Simply Effortless

Style

Lee Heyward

Published by

The Fig and The Vine Publishing, LLC

753 Winthrop St.

Mt. Pleasant, SC 29466

thefigandthevine.com

ISBN: 978-1-4507-9969-0

Cover graphic design by: Cristina Young, C Design, Inc.

Contents

Forward - 1

Introduction - 5

Chapter 1 - Discovering Your Style........................17

Chapter 2 - Shape Up...47

Chapter 3 - Closet Case..65

Chapter 4 - Control Freak......................................87

Chapter 5 - Foundation Creation.........................101

Chapter 6 - The Art of Dressing...........................115

Chapter 7 - Color Full...137

Chapter 8 - Foundation Creation Part II..............155

Chapter 9 - Shop Like a Pro.................................175

Chapter 10 - Keep it Up!......................................205

Chapter 11 - Travel with Style..............................213

Chapter 12 - The Business of Style.......................235

Chapter 13 - Clothes Minded.............................222

Meet the Author - 257

Resolve to Love Your Style....................................267

The Style Essentials List.......................................263

Dedication

To my Mom and Dad, who taught me that anything is
possible...
To my husband, Brian, for his constant love and support...

And to Kristen Caroline, for her lifelong friendship, endless
optimism, and the courage to begin this amazing style
journey.

FOREWORD

My name is Lee Heyward and my job is to make style easy and effortless. I'm sure you read my bio on the back cover, but I want you to realize that I'm really passionate about helping you find your style. I want to reassure you that I'm not that stylist who is the intimidating fashionista. Not at all. I'm not trying to make you runway ready – I'm all about the real world and your place in it. But my zeal is genuine.

Here's a true story about me and my love for style – my best friend can vouch for it! In a way, it's how I got started. I was the girl in the fourth grade who thought a sleepover was a great opportunity for a makeover. Friday night sleepovers usually consisted of two activities: I would either help a friend go through her closet with a mission of finding her "cool" outfits, or we would pour over the pictures in Seventeen magazine and try to make similar outfits with clothes from our own closets. Yes, I seriously was that girl!

In fact, when my best friend moved to a new school that year, my most important mission became helping her to get started in her new environment on the right foot – as the girl who dressed cool and looked great. Who knows how long I spent going through her closet – my first closet edit (which you'll learn how to do later) – before we had put together tons of amazing outfits for her to wear at her new school. I was so serious about seeing her succeed in her new style, I hung outfits on dry cleaning hangers with paper in order to label what to wear with what so she could start her new school stress free. And that's just what I want for you.

This is a unique book – it's a how to manual, a coach, a fun guide to rethinking your attitude, and a good friend who's a style "insider," all in one. I wrote this for you because I know you're busy. You're unique. You're interesting. And most of all, because you are committed to creating the life you want and deserve. This book is made to instruct, inspire, and encourage you – not only to define your own, unique, personal style, but also to make style a really easy, fun, and maintainable element of your life.

You may wonder how you would have time to read this book and do the exercises therein if you're too busy to get dressed stylishly in the first place. But since your style – and what it says about you to the world – is so important, I urge you to consider it in the same way you would any other valuable learning tool or class you need for your work or for any aspect of your life. The investment of time spent with this book will pay off in spades as you'll be able to get dressed and look like a million bucks in ten minutes or less! But knowing how busy you are, I worked hard to come up with a style of book that is easy to read, follow, and – most importantly apply.

About the format:

Each chapter in this book has several elements. I wanted to

break down the idea of style, the defining of style (especially your own), and the styling process into really easy segments full of ideas, tips, tricks, and instructions that will make this an exciting and fun journey.

You'll find Key Points in each chapter. Forget having to highlight or dog-ear a page, because I've done it for you! These key points are ideas or tips that not only help sum up a whole section, but you'll find that perusing them later can help you remember what you've learned.

My philosophy is apparent in the ideas, tips, suggestions, and exercises that are found throughout many of the chapters. This not only helps you with your own attitude, it helps you get to know me as a guide whose specialty is helping you create and maintain simple and effortless style. When you read my down-to-earth philosophies about style, I believe you'll feel even more comfortable defining, working with, and tweaking your own style experience.

So enjoy this journey with your very own, personal stylist in the comfort of your home. Tuck this book away in your purse or briefcase when you go shopping, when you're planning something important, or when you just need a little style inspiration. Utilize it for the very helpful tool it is meant to be. Because, like it or not, style is necessary in a world that will make assessments about you based on how you look. And having style is a conscious decision. It doesn't just happen. You must make it happen! I believe I can instill not only a new appreciation of style in you, but a true sense of self-confidence! Thank you for allowing me to share my passion with you!

Introduction

Attitude Adjustment

Style. Like good manners, style is your free ticket to anywhere. It gets you noticed when you need to be, it sets the tone for the message you're trying to convey, and it is completely necessary – whether you're a stay at home mom or you're climbing the corporate ladder. Two of the many definitions of style in the Webster's dictionary are:

A manner of expression in language.

Excellence of artistic expression.

I like this. Style, in the dictionary, is not defined as you would think in terms of our modern society; and yet those two elements, *artistic* and *expression*, make you see style in a whole new way. I'm here to help you not only redefine how you think of style, but also how to define or even redefine your own, personal style. (And yes, you have one!)

Perception Deception

Style is a simple way of saying complicated things.
~ Jean Cocteau

First of all, let's be clear on this: "Fashion" and "Style" are not the same thing! Fashion can be used to convey your style, and yet, as Coco Chanel famously said, "Fashion fades, only style remains the same." This doesn't mean that style is stagnant – far from it! Your style may change and, indeed, it should evolve. But style, in and of itself, is what the famous designer is talking about when she says it stays the same. This means that fashion becomes a source of inspiration for you to use in order to demonstrate who you are, what you want, and what's going on inside of you, which is, of course, your personal style.

Fashion and style are not the same things!

It may be that you adore fashion, in and of itself, so it's no problem at all to consider fashion when it comes to styling yourself. But if you're cut from a different cloth, and you think you won't like working on your style because you're not into "fashion," don't worry – you'll find that figuring out your style is a fun process and choosing clothing to express yourself can be like an artist choosing paint colors and strokes to create a picture. What is your picture? It can be how you're feeling or how you want to feel. What you're aiming for or what you've accomplished. It can be whole conversations summed into one, concise sentence. But while fashion is something that "goes in and out" and can be bought by anyone, style is something far more personal, instinctual, and enduring.

"Style" is an expression of individualism mixed with charisma. Fashion is something that comes after style.
~ John Fairchild

Some people mistakenly think of style as being rigidly controlled by current fashions. I'm here to help you look at things in a new way. Not only is style way more democratic than that, it is also much simpler, as you'll see in this style book. Designers are merely trying to inspire a look, not force people to conform themselves to exact copies of those fabulous frocks. But it may feel to you like they just don't get you, a "normal" woman of normal proportions. And fashion magazines, while fun and even inspirational, can sometimes be full of empty promises that leave you feeling let down or even perplexed and overwhelmed.

The great news is you don't have to be a devote' of Vogue or any other fashion mag to understand and appreciate the importance of style. And you don't have to be a fashionista to be as chic and effortlessly stylish as the women you admire on the pages of your favorite magazine. You, yes, YOU, can define and develop your own, personal style that says who you are and what you are capable of, both in your business and your private worlds.

• Think style isn't important? Let me ask you this: Didn't you really think about what to wear to school when you were a kid? Especially in middle and high school? If you could realize the importance of style when you were a kid, you can imagine how important the way you look is now when you're all grown up.

You want to know what the best thing about "style" is? It's completely accessible to anyone. When you're done with this style book, you'll be way beyond comparing yourself to an impossible standard in a fashion ad – you'll feel savvy, stylish and confident. And aren't we all the "authors of our lives," hoping to contribute to a final issue that has a little bit of everything, with some fun and flavor besides?

So, whether you're a fanatic of fashion or consider yourself a plain Jane, it's time to rub your hands together in anticipation and channel your inner diva. Tap into who you are and let's figure out how to show it to the world! Let the world know who you are… by your STYLE!

Style is the outer expression of the inner you!

Not all of us are always comfortable with our outer appearances. But your own style can not only be the announcement of what kind of person you are, but the harbinger of potential things to come. Your style can say, "I'm accessible," "I'm responsible," and "I'm terrific" all at the same time. Your style can translate from work to play, from typical day-to-day activities to special events and even to momentous occasions. What you may not realize is that your style is already inside of you. And all it takes are some easy and even fun steps to discover it, define it, and display it!

Once you find a style that feels authentic and easy to achieve, you'll feel GREAT! Let's get started!

Psych Your Psyche

Know, first, who you are; and then adorn yourself accordingly.
~Epictetus

It's all in your head. No, really, psychological studies abound which prove that what you wear and how you look matters. How you look – which in this case means your style – creates a mental and emotional reaction that literally changes how you are perceived by someone or even how you think and feel about yourself. A study by Dubler & Gurel* proved "how a person chooses to dress affects his perception of himself and in that way has an effect upon his self concept." This conclusion demonstrates my philosophy that style should, first of all, be all about YOU.

The famous saying, "You never have a second chance to create a first impression," was utilized in another study done by researchers Biecher, Keaton, and Pollman which found that "clothing helps strangers to identify us and reinforces images held by acquaintances and friends. It's what people see first and remember," they claim, ending their observation with the afore-mentioned first impression quote.

When I help you with your business style later in the book, I'll share some interesting statistics on style impressions in the workplace. In the meantime, before you poo poo the importance of style remember, too, the study by Conner, Peters, and Nagasawa*, which found that clothes literally had a bigger social impression than person and that clothing was a "conceptually important and statistically significant influence on the formation of social impression."

By changing your attitude and then changing what you wear on the outside, you see major shifts in how you feel on the inside.

While it's important to realize, well, the *importance*, of style, my intent is to change not only how you perceive style, but also how you feel about it. Style is fun! Remember how much fun you had as a kid playing dress up? It was an outlet to be whatever you wanted to be. All you had to do was put on a frilly dress and you could become a princess. Or some boots and become a cowgirl. Or a blanket serving as a cape to become a super heroine.

Essentially, when you get dressed each morning, you're doing the same thing. You put on certain clothes and you feel more confident, more a force to be reckoned with, more put together, more modern… or whatever strikes a chord with you that day. That right there is reason enough to have a style you love. If you haven't had these fun feelings in a long time, I recommend playing dress up in your own closet!

The finest clothing made is a person's skin, but of course, society demands something more than this.
~Mark Twain

One of the best things about style is that it isn't black and white. You can interpret style in many different ways to make it work for you. What's important is that *you* are the most important part of the equation. Again, style is all about you. It is the method in which you tell the world who you are, yes, but there are no "rights" and "wrongs" because we are all so different, it's only natural we would all create our styles differently. The point isn't what you are doing or whether you are doing it right; it is about you doing something intention-ally. In fact, that's step number one in developing your own, personal style. Being intentional. But before you can make some "on purpose" decisions about your style, you have to make sure there is nothing left standing in the way in your own mindset.

I really believe that achieving your potential comes from finding a style that makes you feel confident and happy. Then you can pretty much walk out the door and forget what you're wearing –
you just feel good.

Dispense with Nonsense

I don't like myself, I'm crazy about myself.
~May West

There are other obstacles to beginning to find your own style besides the ones I've talked about already. Another one that's easy to get into and hard to get out of is, simply, a rut. It's easy to get into a rut in many areas of life, but when it comes to style, it's like being stuck in what I call an "okay standard." So you're not the worst dressed person at the office, but are you really being authentic to who you are by what you are wearing and how you are presenting yourself?

Think about how you feel right now about the way you look and about your style. If your answer is "Okay" then bingo! You're in the dreaded "okay standard." It's akin to kind of liking yourself, but not loving yourself – or as May West put it, being crazy about yourself. By the time you finish this style book, you'll be so inspired and encouraged that you can have unique and amazing style, simply looking "okay" will not be good enough for you – not by a long shot!

Love yourself first and everything else falls into line. You really have to love yourself to get anything done in this world.
~Lucille Ball

Sometimes lacking a great style isn't so much about being in a rut, but being in a negative way of perceiving things. This is really easy to do, especially since style frequently involves fashion, with its aforementioned outer trappings of thinness and gorgeousness and the like that is challenging to achieve without a personal chef and hair stylist at your beck and call. Even if you're not comparing yourself to petite Kate Moss (or conversely, the gorgeous and buxom Christina Hendricks from Mad Men), you can still get trapped in a negative way of thinking that focuses on lack, or what you don't have or what you are not.

No one knows your own faults more than you do, but there's no need to focus on what you are not; what you need to do is embrace who and what you are. This includes everything from body image to level of fitness to how intelligent you perceive yourself to be. By focusing on your positive inward attributes (like sense of humor, helpfulness, empathy) and outward attributes (such as eye color, lip shape, pretty hair), you begin to develop style that illustrates and spotlights those good qualities. It's not just about wearing eye shadow that emphasizes your pretty eye color – it could be about wearing bright colors because you're upbeat or funky earrings because you have subtle humor.

Self-love, my liege, is not so vile a sin as self-neglecting.
~William Shakespeare, Henry V

Now that you've redefined style – and the way you

think of it – and know the psychological importance of style and have gotten rid of some potential stumbling blocks, it's time to act deliberately. Like I said before, it doesn't just happen, it's intentional. Are you ready to discover your own, personal style?

*Notes:

*The Influence of the Perception of Mood and Self-Consciousness on the Selection of Clothing. *Clothing and Textiles Research Journal,* June 1991.

**Casual Dress at Work. *Society for the Advancement of Management Journal,* January 1, 1999.

Chapter 1
Discovering Your Style

Style is the perfection of a point of view.
~ Richard Eberhart

Think you don't like fashion? Think you don't have marvelous style? I beg to differ! I bet you have at least one or two outfits you love. Maybe it's something you think of as your "go to" look, appropriate for almost any occasion. Or maybe it's a real stunner – that only comes out for something really snazzy. Maybe it's even just a pair of shoes, a purse, or a piece of jewelry. Regardless of what it is, take a really good look at it. That outfit, or piece, is a key element of your own, personal style.

About the look:

> Is it vintage? Ultra modern? Is it sleek and clean? Are the details intricate?

Why do you love it?

> Is it the fit? The fabric? The colors? How do people complement you when you wear it?

What your favorite outfit or accessory says about you speaks volumes! Use it to elaborate on your own personal style by describing it, the way it makes you feel, and the details about it that make it your favorite.

EXERCISE: List some of your favorite clothing or accessory pieces you love. Next to the item, write out how it makes you feel!

NOTES: Jot down any additional notes about details you love when it comes to clothing.

Define and Refine

Fashion is what you adopt when you don't know who you are.
~Quentin Crisp

The beginning of anything always seems daunting. But don't worry, these first steps will be easy. First, you discover more about your natural style. Then you'll go on a hunt to discover what you already have. Later on you'll learn what to do with your closet, how to reprogram the way you dress and all the other nuts and bolts of keeping yourself on the right style track. But as the old saying goes, the journey of a thousand miles begins with a single step. So first things first: Let's see what your style really is!

When you think about the style you want, what words come to mind? Before you answer, I want you to think about it from a unique approach. Pretend you are in a perfect world where you love your body, you can buy anything you want, and you already know exactly how to put amazing outfits together. Assuming this (even if it is a dream scenario), then what words will come to mind?

For example: For me the words would be:

Easy

Sophisticated

Sexy

Unique

Now, let me tell you why I chose those particular words.

Easy – I believe style should be easy. Therefore, every item that lives in my closet helps me to achieve the style I desire with no fuss – it's just easy.

Sophisticated – The word sophisticated resonates with me. And actually I'm not really sure why. However, I know that with everything in life I desire a certain level of sophistication.

Sexy – I didn't choose the word sexy because I secretly wish I was a Victoria's Secret model. To me, sexy means feminine. It means that I feel most confident dressed in a way that shows off the fact that I am a woman and have curves.

Unique – This one is simple. Once everyone has something, to me it loses its luster. I like to be unique. I like to walk into a room wearing something nobody has ever seen. That doesn't mean it has to be weird, it's just put together in a way that makes it unique to me.

Remember, just like the word "style," most words have

multiple definitions. It's simply how you translate the word to achieve style you love.

On the next exercise page, write down your own words describing what you envision (or what you wish) as your style – don't forget this is your perfect, dream scenario.

> *Tip – If you're having trouble with this part, ask yourself how you would want others to describe you. From there, we can translate that into what your style looks like.*

If you're still feeling stuck, check out the words on the next page and circle the ones that describe you.

Sophisticated	Unique	Edgy
Sexy	Fun	Elegant
Personable	Feminine	Kind
Knowing	Easy-going	Polished
Lively	Intriguing	Poised
Chic	Put-together	Racy
Powerful	Worldly	Bohemian
Trustworthy	Approachable	Striking
Sensual	Spunky	Responsible
Unconventional	Beautiful	Mysterious
Clever	Dazzling	Engaging
Charismatic	Classic	Down to Earth
Charming	Articulate	Carefree
Dynamic		

Exercise: Write your descriptive notes here.

Now, narrow it down to your favorite words. Try to keep it under five. Once you've settled on your words, get out two sticky notes. Write them on each sticky note and place one in your wallet and one in your closet. Use those words the next time you go shopping or get dressed for outfit inspiration.

Another great exercise to do that will help you define the message you want your style to convey, thereby further defining your authentic style, is to go check out your closet, your jewelry box, or even the decorative elements of your home. Do you see lots of the same colors? Do you see any themes or patterns (earthy, delicate, structured, streamlined, brights, blacks and whites…)?

If you go through your closet and realize you're really uninspired by what's in there, don't despair! We'll fix that part later; but for this exercise, you can flip through magazines, pay attention to women on TV, and observe women you see out and notice the ones you think look really great. What are they wearing? What do they have on that makes you notice them? Now can you think of some great adjectives to use to describe your own wished for style?

Notes: What items did you see in your closet or home that really inspired you? What were some noticeable themes?

Now, bringing your adjective list from the earlier exercise with you, go and take a look at your closet. Do the clothes hanging there represent the adjectives you've just written down to describe who you are? If they don't, you're not alone. Many of my clients begin with the same challenge.

For example: I had a client do this exercise and her adjectives describing herself included "fun," "outgoing," and "original." But her work wardrobe consisted of clothes that were all dark and conservative. She was matching those clothes to what she saw as the necessary tone to fit the office. She was uninspired when dressing for work because she wasn't being authentic to her true personality in her work style.

There was another part of her closet – the "fun" side – that really did match those descriptive words of her personality. As you can imagine, she was passionate about the clothes in the "fun" side of her wardrobe and looked forward to getting dressed in those outfits. It was like once she was free from work she could finally be herself.

The challenge was how to bring the fun, outgoing, and original side of her personality into her work wardrobe while still making her feel appropriate and professional in her dress. That's just why she hired me. It was easy to jazz up her work wardrobe with just a few, key additions and by helping her to use clothing from her "fun" side of the closet to create new outfits in the "work" side. (I'll teach you how to go through the different segments of your wardrobe later to combine things and make all your clothes do double duty!)

Putting together work outfits in a more purposeful way and dressing intentionally helped her to be just as passionate about her work wardrobe as her play wardrobe. And she felt more like her authentic self at work, which of course helped her enjoy her work experience even more!

So again, the question is:

Does your clothing match the image you want to portray?

Now, if the answer is "no" or even "not sure" then I'm going to add another question:

What kinds of clothes do you think represent the adjectives you used? List some out here.

Do you have plenty of these types of clothes in your closet? If you don't, don't worry, this is more common than you think. For many women there is a disconnect between the style they desire and the clothing they own to create that desired style.

Next, think about what is keeping you from having a style that captures the words you just wrote down earlier. This is really important.

Often there are simple solutions to a problem that's been holding you back from having style you love for a very long time.

Clothes are never a frivolity: they always mean something.
~ James Laver

Exercise: Write down what you see as your obstacles preventing you from having this marvelous style. Or, what would make getting dressed easier for you?

If you've found that your biggest obstacle is simply having a wardrobe that represents your authentic self (which is your authentic style), then you're already starting to gain the tools you need to change that. As you're already starting to see, that's easily fixable. You simply have to be aware of what you want and then make it happen. However, in my experience there are two common obstacles that often hold you back from having the style you want – time and money. Sound familiar?

I can't help you add hours to your day but I've got some great ways to make achieving great style take less time. If you've discovered that you desperately need to go shopping to buy clothes that represent you and the style you just described, here are easy time-saving solutions:

You can develop a relationship with a boutique that will send you selections to try.

You can shop online from the convenience of home at any hour.

You can hire me, or someone like me, to shop for you to find great choices.

These options give you the flexibility of shopping any time thereby eliminating the excuse, "I don't have time to go shopping."

There might be another obstacle in that you feel like

you need an entirely new wardrobe but don't have the money to go buy one. But you needn't feel that way. Often when I edit clients' closets they assume I'm going to tell them to throw everything away. This is hardly ever the case. Usually it's a matter of learning how to wear what you have in new ways, making slight alterations to items that don't fit you perfectly, or determining additional pieces that can maximize what you already have.

Odds are you don't need a whole new wardrobe. You just need new ways to wear what you have or maybe a few additional pieces that can help you maximize what you have.

For example: I recently showed a client that with the addition of one particular pair of pants and a great pair of shoes in a bright color, she could achieve precisely the look she wanted with many different tops and accessories she already had. Far from needing a whole new wardrobe, just two specific items were added and voila' – a new style debuted!

You'll see as you progress in this style book that there are usually simple solutions to each obstacle you face in achieving your perfect style. And it's so worth it to resolve these simple issues, remembering how handy style can be.

Never forget that in addition to helping you feel great

each day, your style can do a great deal of the work for you when you're trying to convey something to the world. Don't let your wardrobe cause you to be a foregone conclusion. Let your style speak on your behalf wherever you go. But don't try to be something you're not or compromise yourself in your quest for style. The fashion industry has a great slogan about counterfeits:

"Fakes are never in fashion!"

Remember that this holds true for you, too! The truth is, that style should be simple and effortless!

Once you find your style, you'll be able to get dressed in 10 minutes or less!

Spit and Polish

I don't understand how a woman can leave the house without fixing herself up a little – if only out of politeness. And then, you never know, maybe that's the day she has a date with destiny. And it's best to be as pretty as possible for destiny.
~Coco Chanel

Now that you have the descriptive words you came up with for yourself and for your wished for style, it's time to get into the nitty gritty. It's not enough to know you're sexy and classic, for example. You have to know how to make sexy and classic work in your real life wardrobe and circumstances. A great way to start with this next step is to think of the following question:

> What area of your life do you have the most difficulty dressing for? (Keep in mind, you're not going into things like "my body style" or "my post-baby weight" right now. We're talking more about the physical conditions of your life than the physical condition of your body.)

Some examples might be something like:

> Feeling like I have personality in my work wardrobe.

> Feeling put together on casual days in the workplace.

> Looking very professional even though I'm in a unique environment or employment. (Like a landscaper, a nursery school worker, going onsite in industrial or construction environments to work, etc.)

> Wearing weekend wear or work-at-home clothes that don't make me feel sloppy.

Working in an extremely casual office.

Write the answer to that question (What areas of your life do you have the most difficulty in dressing for?) below.

Now you know your biggest challenge. To address that challenge and further your progress on defining a workable style, you can answer a few more questions as they pertain, specifically, to where you feel most challenged.

Exercise: Write the answers to the following questions to figure out your biggest style challenges.

1. Where do you go in your daily life?

2. What do you NEED to wear?

3. Do you have more than one "look" required for your daily life?

4. What are some further challenges? (Is your workplace dirty? Do you have a baby and the accompanying accoutrements? Do you have to bring lots of materials with you to the workplace? Do you stand and walk around all day or sit?) List out some of the conditions that can be a challenge in your daily style.

Notes

Congratulations! Now you have some valuable clues as to what may be missing in your current style as well as guideposts for issues that need to be addressed. If you address your biggest frustration (by figuring out how to plan for the conditions of it), then you've overcome your biggest hurdle to creating your personal, authentic style.

Your current style hurdles can become guideposts in creating and maintaining your style!

Re Zone

Make the most of yourself, for that is all there is of you.
~Ralph Waldo Emerson

You're well on your way to simply effortless style. You've described yourself and your ideal style, figured out what types of clothing represents that style, and most importantly whether you have them in your closet. Then you learned some solutions to any obstacles you have to actually getting the clothing as well as addressing the realistic challenges that may stand in your way with regard to your style in general. Before we get to the section on working with your body type, let's make sure there's not one more obstacle in your way – an obstacle that's really easy to miss. Namely, your comfort zone.

Let's be honest. What is your comfort zone? It's what you're used to. What you're familiar with. What's easy. What is so familiar to you, you don't even have to think about it. Do you really want that for your style? Let me put it to you this way. What if someone described you as familiar, easy, someone they're used to and didn't have to think about? That would be terrible! Well, if your wardrobe can be described in the same way, then you need to – as the old cliché says – step out of your comfort zone! And really the word cliché is very apropos here as you can be in danger of becoming rather a cliché, yourself, if you rely too heavily on clothing from that tired, old zone.

Fortunately, there are some easy things to do to push yourself beyond your comfort zone. In addition to applying the words you've already come up with before to your wardrobe and style and being intentional about keeping in mind the things you've learned up until now, here are some tips to get you started on your de-zoning:

1. Imagine you have a friend who needs to borrow an outfit for something. Lay out one of your "typical" outfits you would wear for that occasion.

What do you think about it looking at it from someone else's perspective? If you saw someone walking down the street with it on, would you think, "Wow! She looks great!"? Or would you barely notice it?

Sometimes just getting out of your usual point of view and seeing things from a different perspective can really help you move forward out of a comfort zone rut.

2. Stop taking your clothes so seriously! If you think you don't, then let me elaborate.

When I get hired to help women find style they love, a common theme I see is that they only wear certain wardrobe pieces in a few certain ways. As I said earlier, I will help you to "de-segment" your wardrobe later. But for now, when I see this problem, it may be the result of getting tripped up by the fabric or detailing of a piece. ("Oh, that's satin, so that's only for fancy evening events." Or, "I can only wear that sparkly top to a holiday party.")

The problem is they see a piece or an outfit as a one trick pony. You can work on this by not only coming up with creative ways to wear certain pieces or outfits but also by remembering this tendency when you're shopping. When you are faced with the decision of buying something, you can make sure you can come up with a least a few different ways of wearing it before you bring it home to your closet.

3. Make an occasion!

If you adore something but never have a place to wear it, then make an occasion where you can pull it out. This may not allow your gold, sparkly shoes to be creatively worn in the workplace, but – hey – at least you get to put them on from time to time to go on a date with your husband. Remember how much fun you had playing dress up? You longed for the time when you were "all grown up" and could actually wear fabulous items out in the real world. Well, it's one of the few perks of being grown up. You can! And it certainly gets you out of a rut by giving you a brand new venue.

You can always "dress down" your dressing up if you're having trouble thinking of an occasion. That sparkly top isn't nearly so razzle dazzle when paired with some dark jeans and a cute cardigan…

4. Be willing to experiment.

It's really the most important habit you can get into, both to get out of ruts and to maintain sensational style all the time. You'd be surprised the new favorite stuff you'll find when you just try on something you ordinarily wouldn't think of yourself wearing. Maybe you thought tunics were way too hippy bohemian for you until you realized that the fit of a tunic was perfect – once you found a tunic in a beautiful fabric, you suddenly had a whole new look for yourself!

Experimenting doesn't have to be scary. I mean, if you hate it, you just take it off. It's a learning opportunity. It's not going to change the world – but it could just change your world.

If you try something really "different" on that you love but when you put it on it's just not right for you, before simply ripping it off in frustration just take a moment to stop and really look at it, and figure out why. Is it the shirt's color? That's easy, just get something similar in a different color. Or a different hue in the same color family. Is it the fit of the skirt? Can the same thing be purchased in a petite version or a larger sized version? Does one half of the dress look great and the other doesn't fit at all? If you love the top of the dress and hate the bottom, pay attention to the shape and design of the part you like – maybe you can find a top that's made just like it and pair it with a different style skirt. By asking and answering questions like these, you can start to train your eye to know what you like and what is most flattering for you.

5. Be willing to try a variety of stores and designers.

Sometimes one designer's size is not the same as another's. Even the proportions and structure of the same sizes can be different. Some stores "run large" and some "run small." Just because that fabulous sheath dress at Ann Taylor didn't work doesn't mean a similar one at Talbot's won't…

By adopting a "you never know" attitude, you really expand your horizons.

6. Become style proficient.

One interesting and funny thing about style and fashion is that, as women, we give ourselves such a hard time if we're not automatically great at it. When you think about other things you're well versed in or knowledgeable about or good at, you can usually trace back to the place or process where you acquired the knowledge or talent. And it was often the result of hard work and practice. Why should style be any different?

Chapter 2
Shape Up

A dress should be tight enough to show you're a woman and loose enough to prove you're a lady.
~Edith Head

Body language. You must speak it when you are defining your style. Your body language that is. While you can find ways to incorporate almost anything you love into something workable for you in your clothing, you really have to understand your own body shape before you can make style decisions that involve things like fit, length, and cut. Let's be real. If you adore chunky choker style necklaces but have the world's shortest neck this is not the style for you. If you love a turtleneck but are also self conscious of a large chest, you're only making your chest look larger. Choose V-necks instead to elongate your neck making your chest look smaller.

Now, looking realistically at your body shape is great. But sometimes clients I work with get caught in a common trap. They believe that because they have a certain shape, they are stuck always wearing a certain thing. And often it's not even a style that's actually good for their body shape. I don't believe in pigeon holing – it could lead to you defining yourself as one particular shape. Our bodies are made up of many different proportions. When you understand how you are put together, you understand how to dress yourself in a flattering way.

Great style comes from great fit. Great fit is the result of understanding your body's proportions and dressing them accordingly. The goal is to wear clothing that defines a waist and makes you look proportional on the top and bottom. The visual result is a long and lean silhouette. Who doesn't want that?

Discover your own body proportions by referencing an hourglass. An hourglass is equal in width on the top and bottom. Therefore it is perfectly proportional. It also has a defined focal point, which is its narrow center. No matter what your shape or size, flatter your figure by creating an hourglass silhouette with your clothing.

Exercise: Now let's look at your body shape from the perspective of an hourglass.

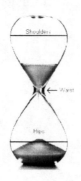

Your Proportions:

*If you do not have a cloth measuring tape use a ribbon and measure the distance with a yardstick.

Measure the width of your shoulders. The easiest way to do this is to take the circumference of your shoulders.

Shoulders: _____

Measure the width of your hips. Take the circumference of your hips at the widest part.

Hips: _____

Ask yourself:

1. Do my shoulders and hips appear to be equal in width?

Yes   *or*   No

If no, which one is wider? Shoulders or Hips?

2. When looking at your shape, is your waist easily defined?

Yes   *or*   No

If no, do you know where your waist is?

Get Waisted!

It may be weird to find out that many women don't know where their waist is.

Your waist is the narrowest part of your torso.

Webster lists the waist as "the part of the body in humans between the ribs and the hips, usually the narrowest part of the torso" in their dictionary. If you take Webster's definition literally, you'll be looking around for your waist too far down. On me, in between my ribs and my hip bone is actually the widest part of my torso. As you are learning you have to take definitions with a grain of salt. Just remember that your waist is the area of your torso that you would like to define, your narrowest area. Therefore your waist is wherever the narrowest part of you is. If you feel like you don't have a waist at all, highlight the area right under your chest which is usually a narrower point for most women.

Apply the Hourglass Image to You:

If you are wider On the Top...

If your top half (your shoulder area) is wider than your bottom half (your hips), you can use your clothing to help your body appear more balanced.

Steer clear of shirts and jackets with accentuated shoulders, as they will only make your top half look wider.

Choose tops that are more fitted and highlight a waist.

Wear straight or wide leg trousers to maintain the balance of your top and bottom half. (If you choose a skinny jean or legging you will only accentuate the fact your top half is larger.)

If you are wider On the Bottom...

If your bottom half is wider than your top your goal will be to balance your body by adding width to your top half. I realize this sounds crazy and I do not mean for you to grab your husband's oversize shirt and call it a day. Be strategic and use the structure of your clothing to trick the eye into making you appear proportional.

Look for shirts and jackets with a more structured sleeve. An exaggerated sleeve or cap sleeve is perfect!

If you are Even Stephen...

If you've already got an hourglass shape you'll find that your top and bottom look similar in width. This is great news! Your job is to focus on defining a waist. Do this with a wrap dress, a blouse with seaming that narrows at the waist, or a great structured jacket.

The Long and Short of It

There is one more proportion you must be aware of, and that is how your body is put together *vertically*. Is your torso long or short? Are your legs long or short?

Determine your vertical proportion by finding your hip bone. Poke around your hips until you find the point of your hip bone. Place your finger there. Take your other hand and place it under your bust line. Does the distance look long or short?

Another trick to this is thinking in terms of whether you are long or short waisted. If you are long waisted you have a long torso, if you are short-waisted you have a short torso. Imogen Lamport, an image consultant, came up with the trick of using the width of your hands to help you determine if you are short or long waisted. She says, "A very quick and easy way to tell if you have a short waist is to stand up straight, and see if you can fit two hand widths under your bust to your waist (narrowest point). If you can fit more than two hand widths you have a long waist, less than two, a short waist."

If your torso is long you've probably noticed that tops sometimes look funny because they aren't quite long enough. Or, when you wear low-rise pants your legs look really stumpy or short.

If your torso is short you've probably noticed that tops are often too long and the trend of high-waisted skirts and pants puts things practically at your boobs.

If you are short-waisted and find that tops are constantly too long, try petite tops. Contrary to common belief petite has nothing to do with your size and everything to do with the height of your torso or legs. A petite top will be shorter in length. A petite pair of pants will be shorter in the rise (the crotch) and in the leg length.

For example: I have a client who struggled with finding the perfect jeans. She owned ten pairs and none of them looked quite right. The first thing we did was to determine her proportions. Her shoulders and hips were proportional; however, her torso was long and her legs were short, something she had never really noticed. She just thought she was short all together. She was choosing low-rise jeans that made her legs look even shorter, making her entire body look squatty. By simply changing the rise of her pants so that they sat just slightly below her belly button, she visually appeared taller.

For another example: I had a client who wasn't confident about her size. She was absolutely beautiful but she felt she had to disguise her body by hiding it under layers of clothing. She wore oversized sweaters and long, flowing skirts, or huge men's style shirts over wide legged trousers. She not only had a wrong perception about how to camouflage certain areas, she also didn't understand that she was making herself appear even larger than she was. Her gorgeous curves were completely disguised and she was so intent on hiding what she didn't like, she failed to highlight what was wonderful about her appearance. While she was nervous about wearing a thinner pant that accented her long legs and a shirt that actually had a defined waistline, once she tried a few new looks, she gained tons of confidence when she figured out she had an enviable hourglass figure.

Her insecurity caused her to make assumptions about fashion choices that weren't the best option for her. And it made her get stuck in outfits that weren't even her style! Turns out she loved tailored men's look styles with pretty, feminine accessories and didn't even like those patterned flowy skirts and heavy sweaters. By taking a chance, having a "you never know" attitude, and being authentic to a style she actually did love, she really began to love her style – and her body shape.

Diversionary Tactics

We all have body challenges and the great thing about wearing clothes is that the right ones can make you forget about the body parts you're not in love with. My job is to help women highlight what they like about their body and camouflage the parts they don't like. To do this, all you need to know are the tricks to dressing for your specific body challenges. Here are some common ways to divert attention away from what you're not so crazy about and highlight what you like about your body.

Look Taller. (Which also means you look thinner.)

• Skip pants with a cuff. The horizontal line of the cuff abruptly stops the line of your leg, making your legs look shorter.

• Choose your rise wisely. A very low rise pant sits below your hip bone and makes your legs look shorter.

• Wear a pointy toe shoe. A pointy toe shoe elongates your leg. Steer clear of very round toe and clunky type shoes, which make your legs look shorter.

• Define your waist. When you define your waist it looks as if your legs are a mile long.

• Don't wear super long tops. When a shirt comes over your butt or past your crotch you can't tell where your legs start. They appear as if they start wherever your shirt ends, making you look short and stumpy.

> *There are many tops currently in stores that are very long. If this is a style you love be sure that your long top defines your waist. This way it looks as if your legs start higher and negates the effect of having short/stumpy legs.*

> *** If you find a top you love that is too long take it to your tailor and have it hemmed to the best length for you.*

• Dress monochromatically. This is a chic way of making yourself look taller. However, I encourage you not to adopt this trick as your only way of dressing.

Make a chest look smaller.

• Choose V-neck tops to elongate your neck. This will make your chest look smaller!

> ** If a v-neck shows too much cleavage, you can always wear a camisole or bandeaux underneath to make it more appropriate.*

• Steer clear of turtlenecks and crew neck style shirts. It seems counter-intuitive, but covering up your chest only makes it look bigger.

• Say no to embellishment that goes directly over your chest (pockets, ruffles, etc.) It will only draw attention to your girls.

• Wear a great necklace. This draws attention up to your face and away from your chest.

Disguise Your Hips

• Wear a wide or straight leg trouser. This creates a straight line from your hip to the ground, bringing the eye's focus to your waist.

• Steer clear of pants that narrow at the knee and bell back out. This only draws attention to your hips.

• Say no to tapered pants (this is a universal tip!) and skinny jeans. A pant that narrows at the ankle will only make you look like an ice cream cone.
• Fit the widest part of your hips. If a skirt or pant is too big in the waist it can always be taken in.

Disguise a Large Derrière

• Do not completely cover your behind. If you want your behind to look smaller, then covering it with a ton of fabric only makes it look bigger. Wear a shirt that stops directly *in the middle of your behind*. Think about visually cutting your behind in half with your shirt. This is something else that seems counter intuitive but trust me, it works!

No Love for Your Ankles

• Skip shoes with an ankle strap. They draw attention to the area you don't love.

• Choose a shoe in a nude color that matches your skin tone.

Create a Waist

• Choose clothing that is structured and has seaming that defines a waist for you. Clothing that is great for

this are jackets, dresses, blouses with princess seaming, wrap dresses/shirts, etc.

~ If you want to disguise a stomach this is also
the way to do it. Remember, your clothes can do
the work for you!

• Wear a belt. Place it at the narrowest part of you.

~ Remember, if you have a short torso be
mindful of the width of belt you choose. A
super wide belt will make your torso look even
shorter.

.

**The most important thing about dressing for
your body shape is simply being in tune with your
individual figure.**

This knowledge will allow you to easily say no to trends that
aren't meant for your shape, understand why a friend can
wear skinny jeans and you can't, and give you a road map for
the styles and silhouettes that are right for you.

Realism Meets Optimism

I hope you already see how thinking of style and defining your style has two elements. There's realism – you have to have clothing that actually works with the daily requirements of your lifestyle, works on your body type and is authentic to you. And yet there's a surprising amount of fun involved – you get to be authentic to your real self, you can try new things with a "you never know" attitude, and with some practice and intention, you can not only have great style, but you can show it and yet get ready for your day in ten minutes or less. I really want to end this "defining" and "discovering" chapter with a key word before you get to the practical applications you're about to learn. That word is OPTIMISM.

Since we're defining stuff in this chapter, why not look at one of the many definitions of that word.

> *Optimism* – A disposition or tendency to look on the more favorable side of events or conditions and to expect the most favorable outcome.

Isn't that a pretty great way to see your daily life? I hope you are getting a glimpse of what having style that you love can do for you in achieving this wonderful state of being. By being intentional, practicing some really easy to obtain skills, and most of all being authentic to your own, personal style, you are, as I said earlier, forgetting what you're wearing and just walking out your door feeling great. That great feeling will translate into all the aspects of your day! So keep that optimistic attitude and you'll find maintaining your style and keeping it fresh to be easy, interesting, and fun.

Any man may be in good spirits and good temper when he's well dressed...

—Charles Dickens

Chapter 3
Closet Case

I like my money right where I can see it... hanging in my closet.

—Carey Bradshaw (Sarah Jessica Parker), Sex in the City

Ah, editing your closet. This is one of my specialties – and it's what will make your life a whole lot easier! One of my favorite sayings is, "It's hard to see your wardrobe through the clothes." Like the forest through the trees saying that the phrase is modeled after, it really can get easy to lose sight of your true style when you've got all kinds of things going on in the shelves and on the racks of your closet. Think about it. How many times have you looked at dozens of things hanging in your closet only to feel, wearily, that you have nothing to wear?

One of the most important skills you will learn in this book is to inventory and edit your closet. It may sound like a pain; but like everything, with the right attitude it can be pretty interesting and definitely instructional. And believe me, if you want to actually enjoy getting dressed and want to do it easily (hopefully with my help in ten minutes or less), it is essential. A closet that works for you is one that is:

1. Regularly edited.

2. Organized.

3. Contains a versatile wardrobe you actually want to wear.

Editing your closet is such an important activity when it comes to finding and maintaining style, I devote an entire workbook to it, do frequent lectures and teleconferences about it, and of course, as a stylist, I get paid to help clients do it. Editing your closet is a wonderfully cathartic thing to do. It's like magic – you get rid of tons of stuff you don't need but end up with way more outfits because of it. How in the world does that work? By getting rid of clothes you end up with more outfits? By the end of this chapter – and your own closet edit – you'll see.

Statistics show that you only wear 20% of the clothing you own. Think of that. If you could have a pile of money that represented all that you spent on those clothes, how would you feel if someone handed you 20% of that money and just blew the rest away or burned it? Wouldn't that be awful? How sad is it to see all that wasted investment?

Well, your time is one of your most valuable assets and with a closet 80% full of garments you never wear, you get a new appreciation for all the wasted time and frustration involved in struggling to find an outfit all these years. Or the time you spent buying things you didn't need or you duplicated. This can happen because you really didn't have a clear picture of what was hanging in your closet or what needed to be hanging there to make your life easier and more stylish. There is something that business people are familiar with which is called the *Pareto Principle*.

Pareto Principle – People only reference about 20% of what they file. My principle – You file things away in your closet just as you do in your work file cabinet!

During your closet edit you will assess each and every piece you own in order to determine what you have to wear, what you need to buy in order to get more use out of your current clothes, and how you can easily create style you love.

The most important thing you need to do before you start your first closet edit is to remind yourself of who you are TODAY.

You will need to assess your wardrobe by looking at your clothing through the eyes of the person you are today. Not the girl of your past, or the girl ten pounds lighter… the girl of today.

So here we go:

What to do before you begin your closet edit:

1. Eat beforehand because odds are, once you get started, you're probably going to want to keep going.

Or, keep a few snacks on hand.

2. Wear something comfortable and easy to take on and off as you'll be trying things on to make sure of the fit.

3. Wear nude, seamless undergarments so you have a clear picture of how something will look when you try on.

4. Have some large plastic bags on hand for separation of items that may be altered, donated, or consigned.

5. Have a digital camera on hand to snap pictures of new outfit combinations you discover.

Get yourself in the mood and make it fun! Put on some great music. Turn off your phone. Order your favorite take out. Send the family out if you can. Get mentally prepared for a few hours of work, even if you're breaking it up into segments. Don't be scared! Once you've done an initial closet edit, it usually won't take more than an hour to do it in the future when you're doing updates a couple of times a year.

Creativity requires the courage to let go of certainties.
—Enrich Fromm

Besides the bags, you need some tools on hand:

1. **Hangers** – If all you have are wire hangers, you need to invest in some new ones because they can cause your clothes to have a funny shape. If you don't have enough hangers, get plenty more before you start. It's no good halting your own progress just because you run out of hangers. Try to use the same type of hangers. You'll also be amazed at how much better you can see your clothing just by having spiffy, uniform hangers in there.

2. **Clear plastic containers** – Storage is useless if you don't know what you have. Clear plastic containers are great for shoes, accessories like belts, handbags and other stuff you want to protect. The important thing is to know what you have and be able to see it.

3. **Stuffing for bags and shoes** – Packing peanuts, tissue paper, or other materials. This helps your purses and such hold their shape while they are waiting to be used.

4. **Sturdy, department store gift boxes** – These make good drawer dividers and containers for loose items for undergarments, socks, stockings and such. You can also purchase drawer dividers pretty inexpensively.

5. If for some reason your bed isn't near your closet, **a rolling rack or something you can set or stack clothes on** is great.

6. **Full-length mirror** – Imperative! You would be surprised at how many clients I work with who don't have a full-length mirror. I literally have to bring one in my car, just in case, when I go to see a client. But style is from head to toe. You need to be able to see the entire picture.

7. **Notepad** – Take notes as you go through your closet and wardrobe. In addition to the kinds of notes you'll read later, you'll need to jot things down about needing more hangers, patterns you're noticing, and other ideas and observations about your clothing.

8. **Written style goals** – Words you've used to describe yourself (remember that sticky note), your style goals you came up with earlier and the like need to be

handy and easily readable as you look into the mirror wearing something or as you put potential outfits together.

9. Another handy item if you have wall space in your closet would be **hooks**. These are easy to find in any hardware store and there are even fancy, decorative ones. These are great for hanging jewelry, scarves, etc.

Note – I have a client who did not have wall space but did have a standing shelf with a long, wooden side that was exposed. She hung hooks all down that wooden side of the shelving and can now see every necklace at a glance. You can do the same in the backspace of a shelf or even a wall if you have enough room. Be creative!

Inventory / Downsizing

At a minimum, you should edit your closet twice a year in the spring and in the fall. But before you edit, you've got to figure out what's in there and get rid of what's not helping you create style you love.

Closet Freak?

Like it or not, your closet is a realistic portrayal of what is currently going on with you. The clothes hanging there are an honest portrait of you when you wear them. So naturally, your closet is a great illustration of what's happening with your style.

I really believe the closet is pretty indicative of what's going on in your life, too. It's kind of like your house. If you're running on fumes and have too much going on, it can get pretty messy and disorganized. If it's not a place you love to go into, then it's uninspired. If it's all jumbled up, then it's chaotic and stressful. If it's neat as a pin but stuck in a time warp, then so is your style.

If your closet is a mess or you dread the idea of going through it, don't worry – it's a natural reaction. If you've been so overwhelmed with style issues (or lack thereof) that you feel like freaking out at even the idea of going through your closet and organizing it, you needn't feel that way. I'll take you through it, step by step. This is so doable! And you know what? It's even fun. I think once you've accomplished this, you'll be so hooked by how easy and fun it is to stay organized and put together fabulous outfits to show your style, you'll be helping friends do it and you'll look forward to keeping it up. So don't be overwhelmed.

Remember this doesn't have to be done all at once. Some folks may like to just save a day and do it all at one time while some may need to take baby steps, having an hour or so here and there until it's finished. But doing the following will help you get your closet ship shape and help you understand what you have to work with for your style and what you need to have to progress forward.

Don't get trapped!

There are usually five scenarios that can serve as traps when you begin all this. Forewarned is forearmed.

1. You don't know how or what to wear with an item of clothing.

2. You are focused on numeric size.

3. You feel guilty because an item was expensive.

4. You feel sentimental about your clothes.

5. You feel an article of clothing is something you *should* wear.

The great thing is that when you follow the directions below, you'll know just how to address (and avoid) these traps.

Categorically Speaking

First, quickly organize your closet so that all your clothes are together by category. Hang or stack all your pants together, all your skirts, shirts, dresses, etc. This will help you see what you truly have. I know I keep talking about mixing things up between segments of your wardrobe and this feels like you're compartmentalizing. But having sections in your wardrobe will help you when you're creating new looks by blending some articles to do double duty later. As you edit your closet, you will address one section at a time.

To begin, choose one section of your wardrobe.

- I like to start with pants or bottoms first because most people have fewer bottoms than tops. Also, bottoms are important basics that will be used over and over to make different outfits so you'll need to know what you're working with.

- Also, be realistic about the number of items you

have in each category. Less is more. Remember that ten pairs of black pants doesn't mean you automatically have ten different outfits. The person who sits next to you every day assumes you're wearing the same pair of pants over and over again. Whereas, three pairs in different styles can actually make more outfits, take up less space, cut down your time on decision making, etc.

• Take notes about color. You'll learn more about color later. But for now, notice what color themes you see.

~ Is your closet full of bold color? All neutrals? All black? Do you have lots of the same color family? You'll quickly see your pattern. You might see all but one or two colors. Or several versions of the same color. You might be in a color rut or might be avoiding a color that you could really utilize in revamping your wardrobe. Jot down your color notes for later!

Now you're about to officially start editing. Ask yourself the following questions about each piece of clothing:

1. Do you LOVE it?

2. Is it flattering?

3. Does it help you meet your style goals?

4. When did you wear it last?

Now, to elaborate:

1. Do you LOVE it?

> Not do you love it because someone you love gave it
> to you. Do you actually love it? Get rid of all senti-
> mentality – this is business. I'm not talking about a
> wedding dress or something you wore on the first
> date with your husband. (*Tip – create an archive
> box or area in another closet you don't usually use for
> those!) But if your deceased auntie gave you 20 sweat-
> ers you never wear or your best pal got you some-
> thing weird from a trip to another country, it doesn't
> help you to keep it. Your closet isn't a museum or a
> scrapbook. It's valuable real estate where clothing that
> represents your style lives!

*If you have sentimental pieces like clothing from your childhood, your baby's stuff, a deceased relative's clothes, etc. take a look at some online businesses that use those pieces as material to create memory bears, quilts, and other interesting items to help you commemorate a person or occasion but still keep your closet for working duty.

2. Is it flattering?

Okay, now it's just you and me here. You need to be honest. Is it flattering to your body RIGHT NOW?

Are you really going to lose 15 pounds by the wedding next month so you can wear your old favorite dress? Do you actually think that your breasts are going to magically shrink so that the buttons don't pull on that darling vintage shirt you want to wear but never have been able to?

Also, in this case, size doesn't matter! Avoid the trap of getting caught up in a number. Just because you can still squeeze into a small size doesn't mean you should keep that skirt if it isn't flattering to you now. Or just because those pants are a "large" size, doesn't mean you shouldn't wear them if they look totally great on you. Besides, you're a sophisticated consumer. You know darn good and well every designer's size is different anyway.

Now, if you're on a legitimate weight loss regime or are still losing pregnancy pounds or something of that nature, there's still a way to do this. Instead of eliminating those clothes that don't fit, you'll relegate them to another spot. But for now you still need to get them out of your "working" closet.

3. Does it help you meet your style goals?

Your goals include the answers to your previous questions. So does the piece of clothing represent your style adjectives? Is it workable during your daily life? Does it help you with your style challenges? Does it faithfully represent what you want to show to the world as representing who you are?

A common trap is that often people keep things just because there's nothing wrong with them – they are perfectly all right, so they hang there, taking up valuable real estate. But even if a piece of clothing looks good in and of itself doesn't mean you should keep it if it doesn't help you meet your style goals. There is often a disconnect between what you want and what you have in your closet. Getting rid of even "good" stuff if it doesn't give you the look you want is a sign that you really are on the way to having the style you love.

4. Easiest question. When did you wear it last?

> This seems like a no brainer, but it really does help
> you make decisions. If you haven't worn it in a year,
> maybe it's not the clothing itself. Maybe you've just
> evolved and it's no longer "you." Maybe you've
> changed a whole segment of your life and your ward-
> robe isn't accommodating that change. Maybe it's just
> not a good fit, either literally or figuratively.

If a piece doesn't answer ALL four questions favor-
ably, it shouldn't make the cut. Be brutal. It may freak you out
a little bit seeing that pile of things to get rid of growing. If a
piece doesn't meet all four requirements, you're probably not
wearing it anyway. All it does is take up valuable room in your
closet and create anxiety when you're in a hurry and trying to
get dressed stylishly. Don't get caught in the trap of having
clothing from the past that hangs on for no reason or that
represents something other than your real life, right now.

* Your closet is valuable real estate where only the best,
most helpful style enhancing items should live.

Your wardrobe should live in the present tense.

If your wardrobe doesn't live in the present tense, that's probably a big reason you may feel like you never have anything to wear. Be brave! Just as a snake sheds its skin, sometimes you need to shed the clothes from certain phases of your life.

Shedding your old wardrobe can go a long way in helping you shed a former life that no longer fits you. That statement isn't meant to make you feel like the purpose of a closet edit is to get rid of everything you own or your identity – that's not the case at all! But sometimes your first closet edit does necessitate going into some clothing and items whose time has passed. I recently heard a stylist named Barbara Horowitz say, "Why is it so easy to consume but so difficult to let go? Why do we think that last year's jacket, like last year's boyfriend, is actually going to come back – or suddenly fit us perfectly?" Sounds brutal but it certainly makes you think.

You should remember that getting rid of something that doesn't fit you anymore – whether that's literally or figuratively – is a good thing. You can still remember where you've been without setting up a wardrobe shrine to honor it.

Also, don't feel guilty about the money you invested in those clothes. You can put your clothes on eBay or take them to a consignment shop to make some money for your new wardrobe. Or you can donate them to a women's shelter or to Goodwill. Isn't it better that someone else gets those things who would actually wear them and benefit from them than for them to be wasted just sitting in your closet?

What is a closet, really, but a catalogue of the different personas we have auditioned and discarded? Hanging there in our closets are reminders, both good and bad, of who we are, who we've been, and who we've hoped to be."

—Tim Gunn

*A last tip is to make note of any easy fixes that would make a piece wearable and able to meet those categories.

For example: I had a client who had a great looking pair of white pants that she loved. But they were too long. She had one pair of extra high wedge sandals that could make the pants wearable but nothing else could give her the height for those pants. So those pants wouldn't make the cut by applying the four closet edit questions. However, by taking the pants to have them altered, she instantly added a summer wardrobe staple that went with all her shoes, as well as her tops.

The Frump Hump

One of the most common style challenges for many women is feeling frumpy. Often it's not that what you are wearing is frumpy; it's that the *fit* of the item is frumpy. Getting rid of frump can be as simple as taking the piece in so it fits you perfectly or just shortening the length. A tiny fix can have a big impact.

> **For example:** Many dresses come with belt loops. Most of the time the belt loops are made of string. Cut them off, which will allow you to place the belt in the most flattering place for you. This can take a dress from frump to fabulous. *Remember, you are in control of your clothes. Make them work for you.*

Can you have something shortened to make it look better? Or taken in for a more chic look? Could just replacing the buttons on a old jacket take it to a new level? Just as a coat of paint can give an old piece of furniture a fresh new look and new life, so can an easy fix do the same for some clothes that you love but maybe don't utilize as much as you could.

The Numbers Game

There's one more thing to consider, now that you've begun your first closet edit. Where is most of your time spent in your life, right now?

Is most of it spent at work? At home? Running around with a baby? Running around meeting clients?

If most of your time is now spent building your own company and meeting clients for coffee or in the home office and your old work wardrobe of somber, corporate suits has been culled, do you have a gaping hole in your "work clothes" area?

If you spend most of your time at work and your closet looks like a boutique devoted to going out on the town clothes, then you need to reassess your shopping / clothing investments and needs.

I'll never forget the day that I never made it to a networking meeting because I couldn't figure out what to wear. Yup, the style guru didn't know what to wear. Unfortunately, I had a huge hole in my wardrobe. I didn't have the right pieces that would allow me to make professional outfits that also had personality. You better believe that has never happened again. I went out the same day and purchased a few pieces that would give me the fun professional look I desire.

You don't have to necessarily run out and go shopping; however, looking at your wardrobe based on what you do on a daily basis will ensure you always have the right thing to wear. Simply make a note for your shopping list as you find items your wardrobe needs.

Ta Da

See how easy? Now, you basically rinse and repeat this process for each section of your closet until your entire closet has been edited. You are then left with a closet full of clothes you actually want to wear.

Chapter 4
Control Freak

Anything that I have ever done that ultimately was worthwhile, initially scared me to death.
—Betty Bender

Let me warn you – going through your closet is only half the
battle. You have to put things back in a particular way so that
you can get dressed quickly and easily. As you put clothing
back in your closet, there are some principles to keep in mind
that will make your life easier while further developing and
maintaining your style.

1. **Visibility** – To know what to wear each day, you
have to know what you have. Arrange everything in
your closet so that you can easily see the elements of
your wardrobe. Visibility is the key to effortless style.
It helps you see what you have so you can quickly put
together outfits and identify items you need. You'll
see some organizational tips later!

2. **Accessibility** – Clothing and accessories need to
be easily accessed. Have a system that works for you.
If you have stuff that is hidden away in unmarked
boxes, you'll never remember what you have or much
less remember to use it.

3. **Flexibility** – Your wardrobe is constantly evolving; your closet needs to accommodate lifestyle changes by being organized and easy to get in and out of.

* On that note, remember to leave room for new additions. If your closet is stuffed, how will you be able to add to it in order to keep your style fresh and evolving?

Hang Ups

There are some decisions you need to make when you put things back into your closet to make sure you keep up the good work you've started. Like how to put things back in, what to fold and what to hang, etc. The key to organizing is simply figuring out something that works for you. (You're the one that has to put everything back so it needs to be realistic for you. So if you're prone to be messy and you're not a good folder, then several shelves of folded T shirts is only going to look good for about a day.)

How you take care of your clothes affects how quickly you can get dressed.

Color Scheme

If you prefer to further organize your closet, do so by color. Create categories within each section of your wardrobe by color (pants, blouses, jackets are hanging together at this point). I do this from light to dark.

White

Beige

Light colors

Deeper colors

Darks

Black

This lets you know how much of each color you have in each category and it makes it SO EASY to find what you're looking for – almost instantly. I mix the patterns in by what the major color is in the pattern. Be sure to keep the type of clothing hanging together. For instance let's look at tops. All of your tops should hang together. They can be further organized by the type of top (long sleeve, ¾ sleeve, short leeve, sleeveless, etc.) Within each type organize by color. So all of

your white long sleeves are together, then your blu
then your black ones. Next you have all of your ¾
which are organized by color. So forth and so on.

The more organized you are, the faster you can grab things in the morning.

* Further tips:

Don't lump short, medium, and long items together. If you have a double rod, place your short items on the lower one. Perhaps you need to add a rod? If you absolutely can't add another rod and have only long hanging rods, then arrange the shorter items in the front and the longer ones in the back, graduating in sizes.

Shelving is a great place to hold knits that would droop or get a funky shape if you put them on hangers. They're also great for T shirts, sweaters, etc. If you don't have built in shelving you can buy great shelving additions at places like Target that can hang from existing bars/rods in your closet.

Shelves are also great for storing your current season's shoes and purses. Remember those clear, plastic boxes? And don't forget to put packing materials in the purses and boots so they'll hold their shape.

* This is important. Create a working section of your closet. This is the section that you regularly make outfits out of each morning. If possible, only put IN SEASON clothes in your closet. Use a guest or hall closet or even a zippered, hanging rolling rack somewhere to store clothes for the other seasons. If you don't have room for this, keep the out season separated in a different section of your closet.

An unavoidable part of style is discipline.
—Tim Gunn

* *Tip to "de season" your wardrobe* — Don't automatically assume that you can't wear something in another season than what you bought it for. Rather than look at what you initially got it for or its color, make seasonal determinations by fabric. You can't wear a heavy wool skirt in the summer. But if your office is cold, you can get away with that pretty cardigan sweater with a light piece underneath it, or wear that jewel toned satin top

with your flowy white pants… See if you can't "de season" a couple of things from your wardrobe to do double duty!

Break It Up

Later in this book you'll learn how to get the most versatility out of your wardrobe. However, the first step to making your wardrobe work double duty, meaning each piece can be worn more than one way, is to break things up. Often it's easy to get into the habit of wearing only items that were bought together, or go together. By breaking them up and hanging them in your closet according to category, you will wear them more.

For example: Do you have a twin set in a great color? Use the shell as a great pop of color under a jacket or a different color cardigan.

To do this you need to hang the shell with your other tank tops and the long sleeve cardigan with your other long sleeve cardigans.

Suits are another item that need to be broken up.

Hang your suit jacket with your other jackets and you can wear it with a pair of trouser jeans for casual Friday.

Hang the suit pants or skirt with your other pants or skirts. It becomes a great basic you can wear with your favorite blouse.

This is a great way to get more use out of what you have but if you don't break things up in your closet you won't remember to wear them in this way.

Congratulations!

You really do deserve a treat – doing your first ever closet edit is quite an achievement! You should be very proud of yourself for not only doing the work it takes to get organized (and in this case doing some very honest appraising in the process), but also really taking a good look at redefining your style.

Restrain and Maintain

Once you've done an initial closet edit, you'll find it easy to maintain it with some discipline. Then it's really just a matter of weeding every now and then, restraining yourself from adding to it unless the piece in question is really a must-have, and being disciplined about keeping it up!

Must Have Habits!

Take care to get what you like. Or you will be forced to like what you get.
—Bernard Shaw

It's no good doing all that work and then losing it all because of bad habits. Remember that it takes 21 days to form a habit. So keep this up. These are things that help you with your goal of getting dressed in ten minutes or less! It also helps you maintain a closet full of wearable, usable things that serve you, and do not impede you in your enjoyment of dressing.

Put your clothes back each evening into the proper categories. If the item needs cleaning, put it in the (properly organized) laundry container. If it doesn't need cleaning, put it back into the section it belongs in according to segment, length, color, etc.

Don't blow your investment by neglecting to care for your wardrobe!

Habit Forming

Some other great habits are to put your jewelry and accessories back up where they belong. Put stuffing in your purses or boots, put the shoes back on the shelf, etc. Don't just throw them in a heap for later. Remember, taking the time to do this makes your getting ready each day a piece of cake.

> • If at all possible, do minor repairs to your clothes that day or evening. A loose button that needs tightening, a stain that needs a soak, a hem coming loose… all these are things that keep that item of clothing from being wearable when you need it. If you put them back in their area without fixing them, you may forget all about it until you're in a hurry one morning and plan to use that item in an outfit, which is frustrating and adds time to your getting dressed.
>
> If you're not a gal who's good with a needle and thread, most dry cleaners can do small repairs, or it's super handy to have a relationship with a good tailor. If many of your clothes need to be dry cleaned develop a system in your closet that helps you get them there. Keep a bag on the back of the door that you immediately put items in that need to be cleaned, that way they are together and handy when you've got time to drop them off.
>
> • On that note, stop treating your clothes poorly.

These are valuable investments! Don't trash your pretty top because you threw it into a laundry load of jeans because you were in a hurry. Use the proper wash settings and detergents. Don't dry if you need to hang. Don't bunch your clothes up in the floor and get them all wrinkled when it would only take seconds to hang them up.

• Quit saving things for a special occasion! This means if you love something in your closet and want to save it, make sure to wear it! Remember we talked about making special occasions? Or dressing something down? If you're not making the most of an item of clothing, figure out why and fix it.

• Stop the thought of always needing something new. If you get invited to something, often the first thought you have is needing something to wear and likely thinking of where to go get something. This is a very bad habit that leads to impulse decisions resulting in clothes that hang in your closet with "no place to go." Obviously I'm not talking about very special occasions, nor of the fun of buying something new. But hopefully with your new point of view, you can GO SHOPPING IN YOUR CLOSET and have a great and guilt free time, too! Just remember to jazz it up or use something in a new and interesting way. You'll feel like you have a brand new outfit.

• Stop doing the work yourself! Make your clothes do the work for you! Having great style shouldn't be hard work – it should be simply effortless. This is easily achieved by fantastic wardrobe pieces that help demonstrate who you are and by using pieces cleverly to make yourself feel great. A dress with a great cut can make you seem like you have a much smaller waist. A fantastic trouser with a gorgeous shoe can make your short legs look a mile long… When you begin to spend your efforts acquiring and maintaining a closet full of useful and smart clothing, the art of dressing will be even more effortless.

• Stop wearing what you think you should wear! Focusing on what you perceive as what you should be wearing can make you feel like you're playing dress up in someone else's closet. By redefining style and defining your own style, by understanding how clothes work for you and how to be authentic to yourself in your clothing choices, you can avoid this pitfall and feel like your own fabulous self every time you get dressed and go out into the world!

BONUS! 10 Habits to Help you Keep Loving Your Style

1. No matter where you are going or what you are doing, create an appearance each morning that makes you feel confident and happy.

2. Kick laziness to the curb.

3. Organize and edit your closet so it does the work for you (like your wardrobe)!

4. Stay consistent with the overall image you want to portray. (So if your goal is to look put together and sophisticated, don't run errands in your sweats.)

5. Take care of your wardrobe as the investment it is.

6. Pay attention to details.

7. When in doubt, remember Tim Gunn's sage words, "Make it work!"

8. Get in the habit of tailoring your clothes. Don't have a bad attitude about it. For the price of a pizza you can have an outfit that makes you feel like a million bucks each time your wear it.

9. Don't settle when buying wardrobe pieces. Everything you buy should be versatile for your lifestyle needs and make you feel great.

10. Make an effort. Small steps have a big impact.

Chapter 5
Foundation Creation

We're all in the business of getting dressed.

—Nina Garcia

After spending so much time in your closet, now is the perfect time to talk about some wardrobe basics. We'll address some more foundational basic pieces of seasonal wardrobes later on. But for now I'd like to help you out by pointing out the **10 most versatile wardrobe pieces you can have in your closet at any time.** This will help you in your decision making about what to keep in your closet. And also what to make sure you have in order to ensure that getting dressed in the morning is an easy experience – any time of year. Keep this list handy to ensure that after every closet edit you still have these "keepers" hanging in your wardrobe realm.

10 Essential / Versatile Wardrobe Pieces

1. **Classic white shirt.** You define the type. Maybe it's a cotton T with a scooped V neck. Maybe it's a classic Brooks Brother's looking button down. Maybe it's a flirty thing with a capped sleeve and a ruffle down the button placket. You define it by your own style. This will go with everything from your work trousers to a casual skirt to your favorite jeans.

2. **Dark denim jean.** This can be dressed up for an evening out or dressed down for a casual weekend. It can even slip into your work wardrobe in certain environments. It's ageless and looks modern and put together.

3. **Neutral trouser.** A great fitting pant is key. Don't forget the length so that it can go with any of your shoes. Then it can be dressed up or down and can be the foundation of almost endless clothing combinations from each segment of your wardrobe.

4. **Structured skirt in a neutral color.** Examples could be a jean pencil skirt, a black A-line skirt, etc. This skirt can go from a meeting to a dinner date to a casual brunch. Even if you're not much of a skirt person, you really need at least one good one. With a simple change of tops, shoes, and accessories, you're perfectly groomed for any occasion.

5. Structured jacket in a neutral color. A structured jacket makes an outfit look more pulled together. This doesn't necessarily have to be a suit jacket. It could be a corduroy blazer, a military style cotton jacket, etc. Whatever you're drawn to will work with your style. Jackets are like icing on a cake. You may look good without one, but you'll look even sharper with one!

6. Camisoles for layering. Why? Black, white, and a few colored camisoles can make a revealing shirt appropriate for the office or can add color or pizzazz to up the interest level of a standard outfit.

7. Tops with color and / or pattern. This is a great and easy way to show off your signature style. Botanical prints, bold stripes, classic paisley… the pattern says a lot about you. And a great color is a great mood enhancer, both for you and for whoever has to look at you that day!

* Tops are so important because they are at eye level. They are also more budget friendly than bottoms and make for very cinchy seasonal updates and changes.

8. Wrap dress or versatile day dress. This is a universally flattering dress and can be gussied up with heels, toned down with fun flats or even really make a statement with some funky or sexy boots. The colors or patterns really make a statement, too.

9. **Neutral leather handbag**. Pull all your outfits toget
with a handbag that's large enough to carry your daily essentials but chic enough to take you from work to cocktails.
Great purses can be expensive, but if you spend your money
on a neutral one, then your investment pays off in spades.

10. **An unexpected accessory**. It's always great to have a
little fun and give a nod to your awesome personal style at
the same time. It can be a red shoe or an unexpected patent
leather belt. It can be a statement piece that really makes an
outfit, taking it – and you – to a new level. If you love something, you can find a way to wear it.

** Is your closet equipped with these versatile pieces? If not, be
sure to add these items to your shopping wish list!*

Down Undies!

Unmentionables – those articles of ladies' apparel that are never discussed in public, except in full-page, illustrated ads. —Changing Times

I always say that a closet edit is the foundation to great style, but your undergarments are the foundation to a great outfit.

Up until a few years ago I wasn't totally sold on that idea, especially the belief that every woman needed a good, high quality bra. During a girls' trip to Colorado a good friend encouraged me to bring $100 with me specifically for the purchase of a new bra. I thought she was crazy. I thought my girls were too small to really see $100 worth of benefit from a bra! Boy was I wrong. I was fitted at SOL (Store of Lingerie) in Denver, CO and discovered that like most women I was wearing the wrong size bra. I was wearing a 34 C and was actually a 36 B. But mostly I was shocked at the fact that I looked like I had lost 10 pounds. In five minutes! Amazing!

Check out the following tips to make sure you have the right foundation.

How to know if your bra fits properly:

1. If your band is too loose you're not getting the support you need. Almost all of your bra's support comes from the band.

2. Your straps should stay up and fit comfortably. They should not be digging into your shoulders. If they are, your band isn't giving you enough support.

3. The cup of your bra should fit comfortably over each breast. If it is too small you will get almost a second boob effect. Put on a fitted T shirt and make sure that the curve of your breasts looks smooth.

4. If your "girls" are closer to your hips than your shoulders you're bra doesn't fit!

5. If you gently pull up on the straps of your bra and can raise your "girls" more than an inch, you're probably wearing the wrong bra.

No Sweat

Sweat happens! If it's common for you, then one of the most important places to consider the type of fabric you choose is your underwear! Wicking fabrics and breathable materials are to be number one on your intimate apparel list for obvious reasons! Don't buy cheap, synthetic bras and panties just because they are pretty. Remember that even in cool weather, your body heat will rise with layers, with climate controlled environments, etc. So your goal, before even thinking of support, panty lines, etc., is to create a sweat barrier between you and your clothing.

* Tip - The difference between wicking fabrics and cotton is that cotton will act more like a sponge, holding on to moisture (even getting soaked and becoming chaffed if too much moisture is absorbed) while wicking fabric is engineered with water-resistant coatings and a system of fibers that move the moisture away from your body so it can get to the surface and evaporate. It's not that cotton's not a great option – it's just that if you expect a lot of sweat, it will eventually be unable to dry out on your damp body.

Chafing Dish

Well, we all know what it feels like when skin rubs against skin – chafing! Not fun! But you might be surprised to find that wearing those awesome figure-shaping garments like Spanx, Smoothers and Shapers, Terri Toners, Kymaro, and others in the "boy shorts" type category really helps you keep your cool while wearing summer skirts! It's perfect just for the comfort of not dealing with sweaty thigh action – the fact that it will be slimming and help your "assets" is an added bonus! Best of all, there are many different price points – they are more affordable than ever and available at our favorite discount stores like Target. Or online and shipped right to your door. To be more comfortable, buy them in a size up so as not to feel as if you are being sucked in all day long.

Strap Trap: Go Convertible

Bra straps aren't meant to be seen. However, it might be very frustrating trying to find a bra that works with all your sleeveless and tank-strap fashions. I believe the most effective solution is to invest in a convertible bra. Be sure you get one that fits you perfectly or it won't work! Most of these bras can be worn with halters, one shoulder tops, strapless, racer back, etc.

* Tip - Don't think that just because you are not "endowed" or are flat chested, that you can get away with going braless. Bras are mandatory, for EVERYONE! Remember that your bra keeps your girls up high, making your torso look longer and therefore leaner. Plus, imagine the embarrassment of nipples poking out or boobs hanging out when you bend over.

Slip and Slide

How many times have you worn a great sleeveless outfit out only to find yourself constantly trying to keep a strap in check? So annoying! First, check the fit of your bra. If it's simply a matter of your shirt not staying over your bra's strap, a tiny and cheap fix at the alteration shop can take care of it. Ask your tailor to sew a snap onto the inside of your shirt strap. Attach a string to the snap and you can keep your bra strap there by wrapping the thread around it and snapping it into place. Some well made tank style dresses will come with a snap already in place. Take the time to do this! It means you can feel comfortable in your clothes and not have to worry whether a strap is peaking out.

Bearing Arms

Not all of us have arms like Madonna. If you're not a big fan of sleeveless and don't like your arms, try to go with a wider strap or tank sleeve, a cute little cap sleeve – or even get a cute, ultra light little shrug, cardigan, or breezy wrap. Don't say no to an otherwise stellar outfit when a quick addition would spruce it up anyway. Also, just try it! You may be surprised at how good you look!

Sheer Panic

Don't avoid those lovely summer sheers just because you don't have a perfect body! The afore-mentioned shaper wear manufacturers often have lovely items that are pretty enough to be seen – or in this case, hinted at through fabrics. Also, a pretty camisole in the same shade as the shirt can make you feel ladylike and sexy at the same time.

- Ditch the "attached" cami that often comes with sheer tops. They are usually a cheap, hot synthetic fabric. Choose something nicer and with wicking fabric instead.

- It's inappropriate at any age, but especially if you're

over 20 – do us all a favor and don't wear a bra only under your sheer top.

Modesty Commodity

A great little camisole underneath something with a low neck can make you feel more comfortable and modest. Or you can try some of those great Bandeaux (extra light weight, colorful, strapless, and stretchy, they're like a really comfy strapless bra but that can be seen).

> • One of the best things you can do to avoid embarrassment or making the wrong impression is to bend over in the mirror before going out. Bend over frontward to make sure it doesn't all hang out (also, press your arms together and move them around while bending over – many tops really gape open with arm movement, showing everything!) and bend over backwards – that short skirt may feel long enough but you might be surprised at the less-than-ladylike view folks get from behind when you stoop over even slightly.

Chapter 6
The Art of Dressing

Zero in on the ordinary thing that you do everyday – getting dressed – turn it into an opportunity for personal expression, peace, and joy beyond words.

—Brenda Kinsel

Dressing for the day is an art. You are expressing who you are and many other things by what you wear. So why do we treat it like a drudgery? Or get into programmed habits that take over and leave us feeling uninspired? Remember, you have your own, authentic style. You've learned a lot already about how to keep it simple and make it effortless. You've redefined style – now let me re-inspire you so that when you walk out the door, your outfit can tell a story about who you are.

When my clients come to me, the number one challenge I hear is that they desire to look more put together. Looking put together comes from knowing exactly how to assemble a great outfit.

Lucky for you, there's a perfect formula to use!

A perfect outfit results from four elements:

1. A key item.

2. A supporting item.

3. A completer piece.

4. An element of pizzazz.

Let me elaborate.

1. **A key item.** How to choose it? Well, this item is the inspiration you build an outfit around. It can be as simple as a shoe, a bold necklace, a skirt, a top – or anything that inspires you while getting dressed that day.

2. **A supporting item**. How do you support your key item? Easy. Just consider what additional wardrobe pieces you can use to complement your item.

To figure out how to do this, ask some questions about it.

Is my item a neutral?

Is it a pseudo neutral (more about that later)?

Or is it a color that needs to be paired with a neutral?

Does it stand out on its own or need additional personality?

Support pieces could be a bag, a belt, jewelry, scarf, jacket – the sky's the limit.

3. **A completer piece**. Now you simply complete the look. In this step you are beginning to put the finishing touches on your outfit. This takes your outfit from blah to hoorah! This is when you make the outfit look like it was meant to be worn together instead of looking like pieces of clothing you just decided to wear together. Again, this item could be a belt, a jacket, a scarf... don't be afraid to plan ahead and try different things.

4. **A dash of pizzazz!** Now we're talking! This is the piece or element that really adds personality to an outfit and helps you make it your own — something unique that defines your personal style. It can come from a special detail in one of the items you are already wearing, it can be an unexpected pop of color, bold jewelry, or a wonderful accessory.

> **For example:** I had a client who loved a button down shirt dress she had but she never wore it. It was khaki and had cool details like pretty stitching, awesome fit, and bands on the shoulders that buttoned, giving it a sort of safari vibe. But each time she wore it, she felt like it was too neutral and she would pair it with funky colored shoes or a purse but it just didn't work. With the formula above she thought about it in a new way.
>
> The khaki dress was the key item. To her, that item said safari. She took off the belt that came with the dress — a wide, canvas affair that was the exact color of her dress (boring!) — and replaced it with a metallic gold and black tiger striped belt she had

fallen in love with long ago but never wore it because it felt like was too much. (She had made a note about the belt during her closet edit to find something very "tame" to go with her tiger belt.) Tadaaaaa! When she put it on her very neutral khaki dress, it was just enough to complement but it had been neutralized so it became part of the outfit. This was her support element. (See how an item goes from "over the top" to "great supporting role" with just rethinking how to use it?)

To complete the look she chose a great look-ing black pump that was a compliment to the belt, which had a black buckle and black stitching on the edging. She wanted to avoid her past mistake of mak-ing her shoes pop so with big color that they wound up competing with the dress. So her shoe became the completing piece. Plus they made her legs look great!

For the pizzazz, she got to wear another item she always loved but never seemed to be able to use. It was a patent leather, shiny, bright green cuff bracelet with a leaf pattern cut into it. Before, she always tried to be too literal with it, trying to pair it with botanical print shirts (where it competed and looked "heavy" in style next to the flowy tops) or with plain white shirts, where it stood out but didn't really "say" anything. The big punch of color she loved was moved to her wrist rather than her feet and the leaf pattern was a fun nod to the safari / jungle theme she had in her head without being literal or cheesy.

It wasn't that the whole outfit screamed "jungle

safari!" Far from it, it was elegant and understated, which were two of her words she wanted to use to describe her own style. But having the "story" in her head and the new formula at her disposal helped her to have a good time figuring out a new work outfit that was transitional enough for going out in, too.

It doesn't have to be even that detailed or complicated, either. She had a conundrum because of a certain piece. But you can apply the same basics to lots of things:

If you're a T shirt gal, then your tee will be the starring role – the key item. Maybe it's got a cool neckline or fancy pattern and a super great fit. Let's pretend it's a fitted tee with a fun black and white pattern. Your supporting piece could be good looking jeans and your completer piece some neutral, nude shoes. The pizzazz could come in the form of a turquoise necklace.

Or go backwards. You have a brilliant, lemon yellow bag that is your new favorite big splurge. It's hard to miss. There's your pizzazz. Pair it with a simple black dress for a key element to ground your outfit, an interesting cardigan for a supporting piece and some classic, red pumps for the completer piece. Since red and black are a classic combo, the red shoes don't take on the razzle dazzle note they otherwise might, they are almost neutral here.

See? It's simpler than you think.

Exercise: Why don't you practice a little by creating three new outfits using the above formula? Keep the formula posted in your closet for easy reference. With a little practice, you'll start automatically putting fabulous fashions together that show off your style! Describe your three outfits.

Double Duty

Now that you know how to assemble the perfect outfit it's time to make sure you are using your clothes to their fullest. This is a versatile wardrobe, meaning that you know how to take one pair of pants and pair it with three tops to create three totally different looks. Basically you are starting to think about how you can repurpose items from each segment of your wardrobe. This sounds way more complicated than it is. All you're doing is taking things from one segment of your closet / life / wardrobe and putting them with other things in a new way.

Get ready because this can actually be fun. You can even bring in a good friend and let her help you and you can do the same in her closet. This is what I call making your clothes do double duty. Soon you'll learn how to buy only pieces that can perform double duty for you when you go shopping. For now, your job is to try and come up with more than one job, or outfit, for the items in your closet.

Here are some examples to get you started:

Take a T Shirt to work.

Use a simple T shirt from your typical "weekend" look and pair it with a smart skirt or set of trousers. Add a blazer, a long necklace, your favorite heels, and your ready for work.

- Please note that when I say T shirt I in no way mean the version you wear to the gym. I'm talking about a T shirt that is fitted and modern. If you are lacking in the T shirt department, Target is a great place to find cute "fancy" tees.

Make a "going out" look sophisticated enough for Sunday brunch.

Wear your "going out" skinny jeans tucked into boots and paired with a great jacket.

Go from work to cocktails.

A classic suit can go to cocktails in style. Take off the jacket and add a bold necklace. Swap out your work appropriate pumps for a great, strappy sandal.

Undo your outfits.

I know you've got at least one great outfit that either a friend or salesperson helped you put together, which is fantastic, except for the fact that's probably the only way you wear it. Look at each piece as an individual and ask yourself how else you can wear it.

Michael Kors says to "Dress up your dress down look."

Why don't you try it? Ditch the tennis shoes and pair your jeans and tank with a sexy little sandal and great jewelry.

Or, conversely, can you dress down a sparkly tank with a pair of jeans for a fun, casual look?

The possibilities are endless. When you get creative with how you put things together your wardrobe will constantly feel fresh and fun. As you create new outfits, don't get tripped up in fabrics. I touched on this before. But here are some tricks:

Satin, silks, velvet, metallic threads, sequins and beads and the like are typically thought of as evening looks. But pairing them with jeans, trousers, and blazers "de-fancifies" them and brings them to a new segment in your life.

On the other hand, tweeds, herringbone or plaid pat-terned skirts, trousers and the like get gussied up with some sparkly fabrics or ultra feminine touches like jewelry or a great silk blouse. Even just making your hair soft and girly with some accessories can up the ante of a menswear look.

Exercise: List out your new outfits you came up with from the suggestions above. Now can you think of some others? How many new outfits did you come up with just by de segmenting your outlook and your closet? Are you surprised at how much larger your wardrobe seems?

Exercise: Now that you've created some awesome and unexpected new outfits, are there any additions that would really enhance the clothing you currently have? Are there some items that are fabulous but still don't have much to go with them? Are there some ideas you got while putting new stuff together to make even more outfits?

> • Leave a notepad in your closet at all times. Make a note anytime you try on an outfit that seems to be missing something. The next time you go shopping you'll have a list of things you actually need.

See if you can go back to your closet, and with a little imagination and some "to be purchased" items, can you come up with at least 2 more outfits using at least one piece of what you already have? List some ideas here:

If you find that your list is more like an entire new wardrobe, don't worry. Continue to jot down your wardrobe needs. For now don't worry about budgets, importance, etc. Just generate a list of what you want for your wardrobe that would help you to have and maintain your fabulous style. We'll cull the list later but for now, just get it all down.

Additional Wardrobe Notes

Exercise: Okay, now take that list and categorize it. You pick how to do that. You can break it up into work / play / special events, into shirts, pants, skirts, dresses, or whatever.

Now that your list is organized, you need to triage each category into three top, most needed items, and then list the items in order of importance. You can even make a "budget for" or "dream" category if you want for more expensive items that would really enhance your style and make your wardrobe shine.

This overly analytical and organized list will keep you on track the next time you go shopping. You'll know exactly what you need and can purchase things that will truly maximize your wardrobe.

Exercise: Category / Order of Importance

Transition Mission

One of the key challenges during certain times in your life is being in a transition phase – like a weight loss program or losing pregnancy pounds while addressing your style, your closet, and your wardrobe. I understand that you may not want to add a lot of "to be purchased" things to your closet list when you feel that in another three months the new clothes won't fit. But I urge you to consider investing in your style during each incremental phase of your program. Of course you don't want to buy several pieces of the same thing. But if every time you go into your closet or walk past your mirror you don't feel like what you have to wear looks good on you and that you don't look your very best for that moment, I really believe it could have even more negative effects.

Having just a few wardrobe pieces that make you feel good about yourself, as you are, can help you make decisions that keep you on your weight loss goals. When you feel good about yourself you are less likely to head to a fast food joint and blow your diet entirely. Just use discretion and remember looking your best and showing your style is always a valuable investment because opportunity is always around every corner. If it kills you to spend money on items you're hoping not to wear in a few months, keep in mind that you can always sell those items at a consignment store, on Ebay, or share them with a friend.

If you're in a transition phase here are a few wardrobe pieces I recommend having to get you through:

Transition Wardrobe Pieces

1. **A bold piece of jewelry**. Jewelry can spice up any outfit.

2. **A casual bottom that you LOVE**. This can be a pair of jeans, khakis, skirt, etc. Whatever is most versatile for your lifestyle.

3. **A wrap dress.** A wrap dress can be tightened as you lose weight and is a piece that can be dressed up for evening or down for day.

4. **A structured jacket**. A great jacket will make you look like you've already lost five pounds and is a completer piece for any outfit.

5. **A few fun tops**. Remember that tops are at eye level so seeing yourself in great color or pattern can be a pick me up throughout the day. Tops can be found in many different price levels so you don't have to feel guilty about getting rid of them once they no longer fit you.

What If?

If you find yourself with a closet full of different sizes, don't be trapped by "What If?"

You've already learned that your closet should only be filled with clothes that you love, fit you as you are right now, and can be used in a multitude of ways. So it should be easy to get rid of everything else, right? In theory, yes, but then the "what if 's" creep in.

What if I gain a few pounds?

What if I get invited to have dinner with the Queen?

What if this skirt comes back into style?

What if…, what if…, what if…. The thing about "what if" is that there is no way of knowing exactly what you'll need five years from now, exactly what size you're going to be, or what's going to be in style. One thing is certain. In five years you will have evolved and changed. Most likely the clothing you kept for the "what if" scenario won't really match who you are and what you want. If you get invited to dinner with the Queen you're not going to root around in your closet for something to wear – you're going to go out and find the most exquisite outfit you can! And if you're waiting years for a skirt to come back in style by the time it does the likelihood of it fitting and you really wanting to wear it are slim.

Keeping multiple sizes in your closet is a little more serious. If you know you are a woman who regularly fluctuates in size, then it is realistic for you to have a few sizes in your closet. Please note the words "a few." If this is a common occurrence for you I would suggest sectioning your closet so that you know which clothes are your bigger / skinny clothes and which ones fit you right now. If you're currently a size 6 and plan to stay there, don't keep your size 10's or 12's. By doing this you're giving yourself permission to have the entire package of cookies because it's okay, you've got bigger pants at the ready. Keep in mind that the woman at size 12 is different from the woman at size 6. Embrace who you are now!

Chapter 7
Color Full

The best color in the whole world is the one that looks good on you.

—Coco Chanel

Are you afraid of color? Are you stuck in a color rut? Are you convinced that only certain colors look good on you, therefore you avoid that color?

Sometimes it just takes a little more information to make you change your opinion about something. And if you've been wearing the same colors for years or if your wardrobe looks a little monochromatic – or all black! – then it might just be that with some new information and encouragement, you may be able to form a new relationship with color.

There are three universal characteristics to describe color.

1. Hue

2. Value

3. Chroma

1. **Hue** – This defines a color's undertone, which is either warm (yellow based) or cool (blue based). Your skin's undertone will be either warm or cool, therefore warm or cool colors will naturally look best on you.

2. **Value** – This refers to the depth of color and a grading of that color from darkest to lightest. This is why you look great in some shades of a color and not so good in others.

3. **Chroma** – This defines the clarity of a color. Some colors are vibrant and light-reflective, and others are muted / dark and absorb light. However, fabric is usually most important when determining whether or not a color will be flattering. Satins and silks (or even leathers or certain weaves of fabric) reflect light, widening you. Matte fabrics like wool, cotton, or jersey suck up light, creating a matte surface and slimming you.

Even if you've had your colors "done" you need to keep an open mind to additional colors that might look great on you. People's skin tones change all the time with change in season, climate, age, even hormones. And you don't want to rule an entire color out that would actually look great in a different hue, shade, or time of year.

Color is a great way to express yourself. It's so versatile as a styling tool also. Take a look at the notes you made about the color already in your wardrobe / closet. Do you see a theme? A lack? An avoidance? Are you ready to have a more open mind about color?

For example: Has anyone ever told you that you should never wear a certain color? I'm a redhead so I was told to avoid pink. But just because some pinks don't look great on my skin tone doesn't mean that

I have to throw out the entire color family! There's a big difference between purpley-pink and a soft, beigey, carnation pink. So think of that for yourself, too. Have you tried a color that wasn't great for you and because of that, you threw the baby out with the bathwater and have steadily avoided all colors in that same family?

Here's an easy thing to do that will allow you to know whether or not a color works for you. Get a mirror and the brightest, best natural light you can. Now just hold the color in question up to your face (without makeup!). You'll be amazed at how your skin seems to transform next to certain colors!

Now I have even better news. You can still wear even those colors that don't look good on you! There are lots of tricks!

• As I said before, there are many different shades of a color. And that means every single color! Even neutrals. That's why sometimes your blacks look different or you can't tell the difference between a navy skirt and a black one. This means there might be a shade that's right for you in a color you previously thought was "wrong" for your skin tone.

• Another trick is to interrupt the color next to your face. Don't be scared of that awesome Jackie Kennedy style sheath dress in a color that washes you out. Instead of editing it out of the closet just put a fabulous Kelly green and cobalt blue scarf on with it and watch your skin shine and your eyes light up! Don't be blue if the funky yellow that's THE color to wear this season is too much for your yellow undertones. Just wear it on the bottom with a more flattering color on the top, or try a bold yellow accessory.

• If the "it" color of the season is not for you, think of a near substitute. If it's all about orange and you look like an escapee from the fashion police in orange, what about a shade of coral that's bright but softer? If mellow yellow greeny gold is all the rage but you look sickly wearing that color, what about an accessory in a shade of inchworm green or lemon drop yellow instead? Remember, the current trends in fashion are about inspiration not dictation!

• Maybe no matter how you wear a color it doesn't seem to work – what if you got some jewelry, a great shoe, or a purse with that shade? That way you can ramp up the color volume in your wardrobe but still look great and feel secure.

Remember, fashion is fun! Play dress up! Experiment and take chances.

Proceed with Caution

Although there are no absolutes with color (are there in any-thing?), there are some cautions with color you may want to think about.

- **It's a Washout** – Skin tone colors like beige, oat-meal, and pale pinks can potentially make you look dreary and washed out. Don't be discouraged though; chances are that there is a tone within that tone than look good on you. There are warm beiges and cool beiges, warm pinks and cool pinks, etc.

- **Black out** – While black as a fashion color is always a hit, its not the best color for every skin tone. There are many shades of black to try – from blue black to rusty black – but if you absolutely don't look good wearing black near your face, remember that you can always just put it elsewhere like I recommended doing with colors earlier.

- **White light** – Believe it or not, not everyone looks good in white, either. If you have a blotchy skin problem, your teeth are in need of a good cleaning or bleaching or your hair is the color of goldilocks, white will only spotlight those issues. Instead of white, choose ivory.

Exercise: Why don't you gather some colors, even if they are in the form of towels, friend's clothes, or what have you and hold them to your face in bright, natural light? List the colors that look the best for your skin tone and pull this list the next time you go shopping:

Myths

There are tons of color myths out there. I'll cover just a few to get you thinking:

• Black (or dark colors) are always slimming or flattering. Well, a dark color does sometimes act pretty slimming. But the cut of the garment is what causes the slimming effect and is much more important than the color!

• Bright colors or light colors always make you look bigger. Again, look at how it's cut and how it looks on you. You might try on something you would have never thought to pick up and find that it makes you look even slimmer than your favorite black trousers.

• You can only wear certain colors in certain seasons. We southerners are especially prone to this – think about the old "you can never wear white after labor day" rule of our grandmothers. Listen, your white jeans might look awesome paired with a camel colored cashmere sweater and some darling, colorful flats in the middle of winter. Your white skirt may become "winter white" with the addition of some black boots and cardigan. That jewel toned, satin top you wore to a New Year's Eve party may look awesome with your spring denim jacket. Don't stick to rules. Just play around and try things. Your mirror will tell you whether or not something works in a new season!

Rules of Thumb

Yes, I know I told you to forget the rules. But you'll find some of these "new" basic rules of style to be more about redefining the tried and true than forcing you into another box of do's and don'ts.

Neutral Ground

Let's start with the world's shortest quiz:

If I hand you a great pair of black trousers and they have a blue pinstripe in them, what color sweater would you choose to wear with them? (If you say you could wear them with practically any color because they are a "neutral" then you are right! If you automatically said "blue" or "black" then you really need to read this next section!)

There are actually lots of neutrals and even subcategories of neutrals! It's not just about black, white, and khaki anymore.

Some neutral colors are:

Black

Grey

Brown

Khaki

White

Navy

Cream

Jeans (yes, as a color and a style!)

Some neutral sub categories are:

Burgundy

Wine

Eggplant

Red

Purple

Peacock blue

Greens

Color combo neutrals

You know that black is neutral and white is neutral. Did you realize that a black and white patterned piece is neutral also? That's right! It's amazing how many new outfits my clients see in their wardrobes once they realize this simple truth. It's not about being "brave" enough to pair a great set of red pumps with a black and white striped dress. I'm talking about putting a bright green top with a black and white patterned skirt or a black and white stripy cardigan over a tangerine dress. You still have to keep your eye out for mixing patterns and not go crazy busy with it. But having an eye for the combo neutrals allows you to keep that creativity level up. Remember to experiment!

Now that you get that, the same rule applies for khaki and white patterns, grey and white, and even black and grey or brown and black – really any neutral color whose pattern in another color is subtle is still considered neutral. Don't get bogged down in the color of the accent pattern… if you keep this rule in your mind, you'll automatically be able to "tell" if a color pattern is actually a neutral. And you'll be brave enough to put together some awesome, fashion forward outfits to showcase your style.

Exercise: Check out your closet. Do you see any "new" color combo neutrals you already have? Can you make a couple of unexpected parings with those items to make some new outfits?

Mismatched

Unless you're the queen of England, then a big fashion rule to remember is that matching is antiquated! Now, to clarify what I mean by matching, it is the practice of pulling exact colors out of a garment and only wearing those colors with it. This doesn't mean to say a monochromatic outfit isn't okay. It's a very sophisticated way to wear color.

When you are fearful about "matching" things, a great way to revisit the idea is to think of nature. There are many things in nature that pair different colors and patterns together to great effect. Think of a peacock, for example. The feathers of a peacock are full of browns, blues, purples, greens, and blacks. You see jewelry and other accessories made with peacock feathers all the time. Even "run of the mill" pheasants are extravagantly colored with good effect. This is not to mean you should go overboard and dress yourself as boldly as a peacock. It's just to get you thinking.

Pseudonyms

Did you know that there are "pseudo neutrals?" While not in the list of normal neutrals above, they are, nonetheless, so versatile, they are practically a neutral. Sometimes it's easiest to understand this concept in the context of accessories.

For example:

A red shoe – Red is a classic addition to any number of colors – black, brown, navy, white, grey, even certain shades of eggplant or green! Probably a long time ago the addition of a red shoe or bag was considered quite adventurous. Now it's a classic! If it would scarcely raise an eyebrow, then it is certainly a neutral.

A blue bag – That's becoming less of a statement and more of a neutral or a classic. A jewel tone, especially in the turquoise family, is a perfect pseudo neutral because it goes with almost anything. You can pretty much carry a turquoise colored bag for days with any number of outfits without changing it out – not because it's "matchy" but because it's more "friendly."

> ** Each season you will see handbags in great pseudo neutral colors. They are a great investment because you can use them all season without ever having to change your bag.*

Look into your closet again. Can you think of some new outfits or at least accessories you can showcase that contain a pseudo neutral element? Hopefully this opens up a whole new outlook about getting dressed.

Pattern of Behavior

Now you understand that you don't have to be matchy matchy to be extremely stylish. You know that there are some surprising "neutrals" in your wardrobe that can be utilized in new ways. You understand the use of color more. You know a great and simple formula for putting together a fabulous outfit to tell your "story" and express your personal style. Next, I'd like to clue you in on the use and mixing and matching of patterns!

Gone are the days when, if a shirt had a pattern on it, it was imperative you paired it with a solid skirt or trouser. You would be amazed at the way you can mix patterns with just a few simple tips.

1. Keep in the same color family.

2. If one piece is an extravagant pattern, the adjoining piece should be subtle.

3. Partnering two patterned pieces with a solid unifies the look.

Let's say you have a skirt with a small stripe in it that also has almost a printed "tweedy" look to it – a very subtle pattern with a few colors, nonetheless. The colors in the skirt are brown, grey, red, and cream but the "look" of the skirt, overall, is greyish. Rather than pair it with a plain shirt (white or cream, grey, red, brown), why don't you try a shirt that has a really bold paisley pattern in it? Even if the shirt has a white backdrop and the skirt has cream in its coloring, you'll find that the other colors – red, brown, grey – are a unifying element. The bold shirt gives the more subtle skirt some sparkle, if you will. Put a brown or red or grey cardigan over it, and you have a really snazzy, interesting look that manages to look smart without seeming overdone.

Or let's take your black trouser with the blue pin stripe mentioned before. If you paired that with a shirt that had a bold circular pattern of red, blue, black, and white, your outfit will be more fun and winsome rather than being boring with the pairing of a blue button down top with a black cardigan.

If you're still not sold, think about a man wearing a suit. A well dressed man can be found wearing a pin stripe suit with a striped shirt, patterned tie, and possibly even a pocket square. The reason this works is that there is typically only one pattern that your eye is drawn to, whether it is the shirt or the tie. The rest of the patterns add an interesting touch to an outfit that simply goes very well together.

Again, just experiment with an open mind. If you hate the combination, or it really does seem too busy, just take it off. But you just may find a new favorite outfit that makes you look stylish and confident rather than safe and boring.

Chapter 8
Foundation
Creation Part II:
Seasonal Successes

Ah, summer, what power you have to make us suffer and
like it.
—Russel Baker

Now that we've inventoried and edited your closet and gotten
some of the fundamental basics needed in every wardrobe,
this would be a good time to recommend some seasonal
basics for you. If you have some basics for each season, then
you can infuse your own special touches and some new trends
throughout the year to keep your style fresh and interesting.

In the fashion world there are two main seasons:
Spring and Fall.

Let's first take a look at what I will call your Spring/Summer
season. We'll start with some key pieces.

Key Pieces for Spring/Summer

White jean

Easy dresses

Printed Blouse

Trench Coat

Lightweight Cardigan or Jacket

Shorts

Denim Skirt

Sunglasses

Bathing Suit

Bathing Suit cover up

Fancy Tees

Ballet Flat

Wedge Sandal

Fancy Flip Flop

In the summer the fabric you choose can make or break how comfortable you are. Choose natural fabrics for warmer weather like:

Cotton

Silk

Linen

Lightweight wool (yes, there are types of wool that are very breathable and don't absorb sweat!)

Technological fabrics. Remember these from our underwear section? It's not just for workout clothes anymore as more manufacturers are using "wicking" materials in more and more ways!

Tip: Remember what wicking fabric is? It literally "wicks" or absorbs moisture away from the skin. The fabric is engineered with water resistant coatings and a system of fibers that help to move the moisture away from the body.

Some companies that use these fabrics in fashion forward ways include:

Bamboosa

Lifestyle sections of athletic companies like Adidas, Columbia, etc.

Prana

Athleta

Columbia

We've addressed many summer related wardrobe issues in the underwear section. But here are some extra issues you may be wondering about when it comes to the basics of dressing for the hot season.

Short Cuts

Shorts. They get a bad rap and they shouldn't! I believe there is a pair of shorts for everyone – or at least a way to get the look of shorts for any body type. Even if you think, "I don't do shorts!" it's pretty hard to get through the entire summer without some. It's best to go ahead and figure out what works for you and have some handy if you're serious about beating the heat in style.

Shorts are really versatile – shorts paired with heels

can be surprisingly elegant. Shorts can be skirtish, flirty, feminine, tailored, dressy, casual… Everything a pant can be.

But there are elements to be concerned with also – shorts
can be:

Too big

Too small

Too short

Too long

Too hoochie mama

Too wild

Too conservative

And often there's a very fine line between those elements.
Sexy becomes hoochie when the heel's too high and the
short's too short. Preppy becomes boring when paired with a
manish button down. But once you get the right short in the
right fit, you can build outfits that really showcase your style.

The trick to shorts is easy – to find a pair that shows
off the good and camouflages the bad. Think about your
favorite pair of trousers. They probably have a fairly straight
leg and create a vertical line from your hip to the ground.

Your favorite pair of shorts should do the same thing. It's just a matter of finding the right fit for you.

And please don't think you can't show your legs! No one's legs are perfect! Not even models' legs are perfect – what do you think airbrushing is for? Since we don't have the benefit of such an insta-fix, we must work with what we got. There are great products out there to boost your shorts self esteem, too. Instant tanners, cellulite smoothing creams, wonderful hair removal products, firming agents, even makeup for scars, veins, and blemishes. Keep an open mind if you're normally "not into" shorts. And be careful in your shorts choices. Just because they are a more casual item of clothing doesn't mean you can choose carelessly or forget that these, too, are indicative of your own, personal style.

When looking for shorts, look for three things:

1. Length

2. Shape

3. Versatility

1. **Length** – It's essential you find the right length for you (not what's currently "hot"). You'll base this length on the

shape of your leg and your height.

> If you are SHORT – your shorts should be shorter. Long shorts will make your legs look even shorter. (That doesn't mean daisy dukes are in!)

> Longer legs have a little more versatility – but short shorts might lead to a spindly, spider leg look.

> Length can also be determined by the next element, shape.

2. **Shape** – Your thigh shape is important when it comes to shorts. Your thigh is not a rectangle or a circle. It's a unique shape that will narrow and widen at certain points of your leg.

> A good rule of thumb is that the length should stop at the point where your leg looks the slimmest. Remember that you are in control of this. Stand in the mirror and play with the hem until you find the right length for you.

> Experiment with it! Have fun!

3. **Versatility** – A tailored short in a neutral color can be

worn in endless ways. They can be dressed up with a wedge or down with a flip flop. A neutral fabric helps in flexibility.

A crazy print or loud color may make you think "Yea! Summer's here!" But you can only create a couple different looks with those. You want a short that will go with tons of tops and shoes, not a one hit wonder!

Also remember that like any other outfits, shoes can make or break a look for your shorts' style. It's not that you have to get fancy with it. A cool, fashion forward sneaker or sandal can make a great statement about you. My personal favorite shoe to pair with shorts is a great wedge sandal.

And a shoe can elongate the look of your legs, too! A neutral color shoe really helps with this. Think of how long your legs would look in a tan shoe with a cork wedge! My own Cole Haan pink shoes are a great neutral for me because of my skin tone. Experiment with your own neutrals to see what makes you long and leggy.

Flip Flops

During the summer it's easy to live in flip flops. However, I remind you to take care of your feet. While no style of shoe is off limits (except maybe at work), beware of wearing a certain type of shoe day in and day out – especially if it does not have the support you need.

For example:

An endless shoe wardrobe of flip flops doesn't give your feet the support they need. Your foot can actually spread and widen with heat and stress!

A shoe with no back makes your foot work extra **hard** just to keep it on – even if you don't feel it. This puts a big strain on the muscles that run on the bottom of your foot. Even a tiny strap can make a big **difference.** Stick with what I call a fancy flip-flop which is a stylish flat sandal that has some support for your feet.

Try Sofft shoes. They have fabulous styles with comfort and support as a first priority! Let's face it. Your shoes might rock the house, but if you're feet are killing you within minutes, you are not going to present your best self to those around you.

Teed Off

T shirts are not what they used to be! Look into getting some fabulous fancy tees and watch them go from day to night by switching a cool canvas sneaker to a sexy wedge sandal – same shirt, same shorts, new outfit. Now that's repurposing.

Remember what we said about a fancy tee? Great color, great fit (forget the boxy boy look!), groovy design on it, or embellishments like stitching, interesting neckline, even sparkles. They're available everywhere and are such a great bargain.

Easy Dresses

Don't think you're just not a "dress girl" because dresses are so versatile. A great pattern can carry your style look forward in a huge way. A neutral shade lets you really play with your accessories and transition from event to event. Quirky additions like a lightweight scarf, belt, or even a cardigan can further shake it up. Dresses can be dressed up and down and are a summer wardrobe staple.

Key Pieces for Fall / Winter

Leather Jacket

Neutral ¾ Length Coat

Interesting Sweaters

Neutral Cardigan or Jacket

White or Black Turtleneck or
Crewneck Tee for layering

Tweed Skirt

Fun lightweight scarf

Pashmina in bold color

Dark Denim Jean

Neutral Wool Trouser

Boots

Patterned Hosiery

Layering

Layering is a must for warmth in the winter. However, if it's done wrong you end up looking like the Michelin Tire man. Stick to thin layers that look neat and smooth underneath your clothes. A great way to make your favorite dress more winter appropriate is to wear a turtleneck or long sleeve crewneck underneath. Or combat the chill of the wind by wearing a camisole underneath your favorite sweater.

Socks/Hosiery

Nothing kills an outfit like the wrong sock, in particular an athletic sock. Upgrade your socks to thin trouser socks. Your socks should match your pants.

And speaking of what goes on your feet, hosiery has come a long way. There are tons of colors and patterns of panty hose and tights. Don't be afraid to experiment. For a more subtle look choose a patterned tight/ hose in a similar color to your skirt of dress. For a bold look wear a contrasting color tight such as black with a white skirt, or maroon with a grey dress.

Detailed Sweaters

If sweaters are a mainstay for your fall and winter wardrobe be sure to choose ones with visual interest and detail. Nothing slows down a morning like trying to add pizzazz to a boring solid V-neck sweater (and if your closet is already full of these, try them with a bold scarf or fun brooch). Look for sweaters with interesting embellishment, pattern, or great color. It can really add some excitement to a dreary winter day.

Fitted Outerwear

A wardrobe mistake that I see over and over again is outerwear that is too big or has no shape. Yes, you need to buy your winter coat so that it comfortably fits over a typical winter outfit but make sure it has a fitted and flattering silhouette. You can even add a belt to your winter coat to improve the fit and give it more of a style statement.

Transition Season

While there are four seasons in the year, there are really two transitions when it comes to expressing your style through your wardrobe. Spring and Fall can be very challenging in most regions of the country.

There are usually three challenges to transition times:

1. You're not sure of the rules you should follow about what you can and cannot wear.

2. You are bored with your current season's wardrobe and want to start experimenting in the new seasonal trends.

3. You want to start updating your wardrobe to continue feeling fresh but aren't sure which new styles are ones you can wear now and throughout the season.

It's not always easy to transition from one season to another wherever you may live. If you live in the south, it gets tricky when the stores are full of wool and faux fur, sweaters and boots, but the thermometer still reads above 80°. While the sun is still scorching coastal cities, bathing suits go missing on boutique racks in order to make room for the heavy winter wear. While in the northern region and climes, light and springy fabrics bring bursts of fresh color but not the warm necessities shoppers need while they are still bundled up against still-low temperatures that are typical of spring and early summer. Then you have the challenges of climate-controlled environments. The air conditioning at work and in public buildings makes it feel like winter, so that adorable sundress offers little comfort. Or the heat in the same places during the winter causes you to sweat profusely in your wonderful new cashmere sweater and groovy boots.

But there are easy ways to infuse your wardrobe with seasonal trends and still deal with the realities of your climate – and climate controlled environments.

The easiest tip is to wear the "in" colors of the season in fabrics that are appropriate for where you live. Maybe you can find that splendid fall plaid in a light cotton skirt or jacket for a hot September in the lower south.

Conversely, a twin sweater set in a gorgeous, bright spring hue might be just the thing for a very chilly early May in New England.

Another thing to remember is to pay attention to the fabrics that are traditionally indicative of a season.

* Eyelet, seersucker, gauze, linen, straw, etc. scream summer no matter what color they are.

Tweeds, wool, velvet, suede and the like are more typical in the fall and winter.

But some fabrics are fabulous at doing double duty, like denim - White jeans can look awesome in fall or winter paired with boots and a great jacket. And even the darkest denim does just fine with a skimpy tank and some summery flip flops in the warm season.

Arm's Length

A great way to play with a new season is sleeve length. Just a simple change up to an elbow length sleeve from a short sleeve or tank is a great way to segway into a more fallish look. Or what about paring a tank top with another layer of something with a long sleeve?

Leg Up

While it's pretty easy to get away with any length of sleeve in transitional times, pants are a different matter. If you're truly wanting to look "fall" then you never will while wearing shorts or capris! If it's too hot for pants, go with nice skirt instead with a fall look or color. And you may put a sweater with shorts but it's still going to look like a summer look trying to wedge its way into winter.

Hoofin' It

Shoes are great way to transition into a new season. Pair the jeans, tank, and light jacket you would have worn in summer with some darling velvet or sued flats or short boots and you have instant fall. Ditch the loafers for some cool cork wedges or a bright, strappy sandal and your classic wide legged trousers gain a light, springy feel. Take advantage of those types of shoes that bespeak a specific season. Sandals and flip flops are summer all over. Boots are great to transition into fall.

* BUT NEVER FORGET NOT TO GET BOGGED DOWN IN THE RULES!

When to buy Seasonal Updates:

Many times the seasonal key pieces you desire aren't readily available during the exact time in the season you want them. This is particularly the case if you live somewhere where the climate has a lengthy transition season. It's good to keep an eye out for the items you need based on stores annual merchandising schedule. This way you will have the best selection.

January – Spring Jackets

February / March – Denim

April – Bathing Suits and Summer Shoes

May- Shorts/ Summer dresses

June – Dresses/ Tanks

July – Lightweight sweaters and long sleeve tees

August – Winter Coats and boots

September – Boots

October – Sweaters and holiday

November – Holiday / gifts

December – Resort items

Chapter 9
Shop Like a Pro

If men liked shopping, they'd call it research.

—Cynthia Nelms

Make Great Style Happen!

Last chapter you learned to be ruthless when you were editing your closet. You have to do the same thing when you shop! Shopping is an intergral part of creating style you love. When you shop you are purchasing items that you use to create style you love. Duh! However, as simple as that concept may seem most wardrobes get derailed at the store. This chaper is designed to give you tools and direction to make your shopping successful and fun.

Habit Forming

Think about your current shopping habits. Here are some questions to ask yourself to get a realistic look at how you shop:

1. What motivates you to head to the store?

2. When you make a purchase, do you end up with items that help you change the feeling that you have nothing to wear?

If you answered yes to the second question, congratulations! That means all the difference between shopping and shopping successfully.

When you shop successfully, your purchases can immediately be integrated into your existing wardrobe and will also help you fill a need within your wardrobe.

Meeting your Needs

What is a need in your wardrobe? It's like a hole that needs to be filled. It's simply something you don't have that you could really use (hopefully from your lists and ideas from your closet edit). When you figure out what your needs are, you have priority items on a list that you can shop for rather than just going in for a one trick pony outfit or worse, just wandering around making impulse purchases.

* Tip: Remember that everything you buy should perform double duty.

This is a great place to "triage" – that is, to choose the top three needs you CURRENTLY have in your wardrobe. Maybe you realize you need some transitional items for the new season. Maybe you're in a new job and your wardrobe is way too formal and you need to find some more dressed down items. Maybe you have no pretty sweaters and it's all sweatshirts on your shelves. It's a great idea to write down your top needs before doing any of the following prep work for shopping.

Before we hit the stores, let's go a little deeper into what makes us tick when it comes to shopping and buying.

Why Buy?

Let's talk some more about WHY you shop.

1. You have a need. Something is missing from your wardrobe – that hole we spoke about – and that something is what you need to accomplish your style goals.

2. You want something. It may be something you have had your eye on or is on your list. But here I'm speak-

ing about wanting something emotionally.

There's something fun about getting something new! If you like to shop, you are often emotionally driven to buy things. This is where a lot of those items in your closet that you bought and never really wore came from. Don't worry, it happens to all of us at one time or another.

3. You are bored and shopping is something to do. It's entertainment. Don't worry if you feel this way – it's actually how I started my career.

I was working as an equestrian footwear and apparel sales rep and traveled a lot. I loved the job, but that meant at night I was looking for something to do. So to the mall I would go. I spent five years shopping out of boredom! I got some great stuff but I also ended up with tons of things I didn't need, as you can imagine. It taught me a lot that added to my passion for style. You never know where you'll get that future career training!

4. Shopping can also be a social activity. It's a great thing to do with friends and family.

Shopping nowadays has become an experience and a source of entertainment. The swank places make you feel like royalty and the discount stores and sales at department stores make you feel like you got away

with something with their fabulous bargains. (Just remember, it's not a bargain if you never wear it!) Many
places you shop now also have other "experiences"
to offer you in addition to shopping. You can have
coffee, eat, hang out… and there's a great reason they
want you to linger in there. It's not about hospital-
ity – studies show that most actual sales occur in the
third hour of shopping! That's why malls and such
are designed to keep a shopper there for at least that
amount of time. Fountains, cool architecture, music,
and other bells
and whistles contribute to your experience to get you
to stay.

While all this seems to complicate the activity (or the
art?) of shopping, there are three easy things to remember
that will help you obtain your style goals while avoiding shopping traps.

You have to:

1. Have a plan.

2. Be disciplined and discriminating.

3. Be willing to simply try something on.

Now, let's elaborate.

1. **Having a plan** – To illustrate this first point, I'll tell you about my love / hate relationship with the grocery store. I would say that I'm grocery store "challenged." I know there are all these yummy ingredients that, when combined together, will make a fabulous meal. But I have no idea what to get. So I end up getting the same items over and over and then feel sad at home when I have nothing special or inspiring to make.

The same thing happens with your clothes. When you go shopping without a plan and without paying attention to what you're doing and what your goals are, you probably tend to go to the same stores. Without realizing it, you may be bringing home items that are very similar to what is already hanging in your closet. It's time to break that pattern! Here's where having a plan comes in. Rather than just jumping in the car and heading to the store, just take the time to do a little legwork. Here's how to have, stick to, and even enjoy your shopping plan:

> Check out your closet. Remember what you have and what you need. This is a good time to check your priority, "for-right-now" list that is hopefully triaged. You'll be amazed at how much calmer you are when you already know what you're going for and don't have the pressure of getting a whole new outfit.

Put on clothing that is really easy to get on and off.

> ** Remember that too much makeup will be a pain when you're slipping things over your face. But not enough and you won't feel pretty and confident so you might not like anything you find.*

Make sure you're wearing comfy shoes. Who wants to walk around with sore feet all day? They need to be easy to get on and off, too.

Gather any items you want to bring along with you to match up additional pieces with, to make sure of color, etc.

Bring your calculator! This will really help you stick to your budget and compute your CPW's for potential garments. Don't worry, you'll learn what a CPW is in just a moment!

Jot down your overall style goals – or at least some-thing that helps you remember them. This really does help. If your style goals include more work pieces and dressing up your dressed down look, then you can avoid buying yet another T shirt just because it's on sale or another pair of jeans just because they're a fabulous price.

Put on a positive outlook. This is especially important if you don't like to shop or are feeling like you have an awful lot of wardrobe "fixing" to do after your first edit. Just remind yourself about things that may bug you: Not everything is going to fit. It will take some time to make intelligent and interesting choices. If something you love on the rack just doesn't work, there's something else out there that will.

You wouldn't put together a bid package without a little prep work. You wouldn't meet a new client without your ducks in a row. You wouldn't leave the house with your baby without a bag full of what you need on an outing. Why would you expect to have success shopping for new wardrobe pieces without getting your act together first? This preparation will more than pay for the time invested because it will make shopping so much easier and more relaxed. And your wardrobe will be enhanced with even more style showcasing items.

2. **Be disciplined and discriminating** – This sounds like a no brainer, but you really have to keep this in mind. It's actually the most difficult part of the style equation. For many of the reasons you've already learned about and will ahead, it's really easy to get distracted or even derailed when you go shopping. Consuming is fun, but it's even more fun when it's guilt free. Making sure you don't come home with something you already have enough of or doesn't help you with your holes and your style goals will certainly help you out in the guilt free department. There are three rules to remember to

being disciplined when shopping.

A deal isn't always a deal.

Remember that statistic where you only wear 20% of what's in your closet? Well, so called bargains are often the impetus to this. If your biggest hole in the wardrobe is more trousers for work, then it doesn't matter how cheap that designer dress is, you won't make good use of it. Those black pants may be marked off 60% but if you already have three pairs, why do you need yet another?

An item should work double duty.

I'll go ahead a put a disclaimer on that and say yes, there are occasions that you may need an item that's only worn once. But I'm not talking about a special event. When it comes to most articles of clothing, they need to be versatile, mix with what you already have, and also go from one section of your closet to another and be dressed up or down or used in a few ways. As for the special event stuff, with some careful thought and a little work at the store, you may surprised that you can actually pick out something you can use again.

Your body isn't the enemy.

That may sound funny, but what's not funny is finding

shopping really frustrating because of body issues and challenges. But listen, it's not your fault if something doesn't fit you right. Remember, companies use fit models who are very proportional to make a pattern for their clothing sizes to go off of. The challenge there is that we are all totally different sizes and proportions. Those people you feel look perfect are only very good at hiding their flaws because there's no such thing as a perfect body. Every body is naturally asymmetrical. One breast is larger, one shoulder is higher, one leg is longer. Some brands and cuts simply might not work for your body shape while others will. This goes back to a lesson you learned in your closet edit – the one where you only buy things that fit you as you are right now. That present tense wardrobe, remember?

3. **Be willing to try things on** – The old try before you buy adage works here. First, trying something on ensures you don't make a purchasing mistake. People often believe they will take something back if it doesn't work and then wind up hanging onto it – taking up valuable closet real estate. Secondly, the act of taking it to the changing room and trying on buys you a little time. When you have a little practice being a disciplined shopper, you'll often realize during the time it takes to do all this that you really don't need this item after all. You ensure it's really what you're looking for and not an impulse decision. I know this seems funny and obvious, but it's really one of shopping's golden nuggets of wisdom.

You really have to be certain that an article either fits perfectly already or can with a little alteration. And be honest with yourself. Will you really take a garment to the alteration shop or will it just hang in your closet taking up space?

Have a Fit

Since you now know you have to try EVERYTHING on, you'll find some common issues with size and fit. It's important to know which ones can be altered and when you need to try again. See if any of these sound familiar.

Spill over – If anything is pinching, cutting, stopping your circulation, or pushing things where they don't need to go, it doesn't fit and it's not worth it to buy that item. There are some instances where this can be fixed – like a sleeve whose arm is too tight that has a button or tab on it that can be altered. But issues like the famous "muffin top" on jeans simply can't be fixed. The "muffin top" comes from a waistband that is simply too tight. Try going up a size or finding a pant that hits you in a different part of your torso, such as slightly higher or lower.

A poor fitting crotch – Extra fabric that sags around the crotch isn't ladylike. Frankly, you'll wind up looking like a man. Or the opposite can also happen. You spend your whole day scootching around and pulling on your bottoms because the crotch is too short – or worse, you get the infamous look of a certain desert animal in a certain place. Not acceptable. If the crotch doesn't fit look for a different pair of pants.

A skirt or dress is too tight in the hips – If the fabric around your hips is too tight, even just a bit, it will wind up pulling across your crotch. It creates a few horizontal wrinkles that indicates to anyone that the fit isn't right. And it looks messy. Remember that you have to fit the widest part of you first and if the waist ends up being too big you can always take it in.

Too tight across the chest – If a top is too tight across the chest it will do the same thing, making horizontal wrinkles. If a blouse buttons, it needs to close all the way without having any pulling or gaps between the buttons. Now, if you have a very slight gap (and I do mean slight), this might be something you can fix with fashion tape, which is double-sided tape that won't mess up your clothes. Or, by having a very small button put in at the place of the gap.

Panty lines – There's nothing worse than this – what an easy way to mess up your whole look. But if you're not a thong fan, that's okay. There are plenty of styles that work really well and do not show panty lines. Just remember, before you leave the house in the morning, turn around and check your hiney in the mirror!

Gaping Waistband – This happens especially on women who are curvy but have a small waist. It's a real pain because you have to try on what feels like a million pairs of pants to find the ones that don't show your underwear when you sit down or bend over. While there are different cuts and styles that help combat this often the solution is simply having to fit the widest part of your body and then have the waist of your pants taken in. Do it! A $20 investment might really take your wardrobe to a new level with an awesome fitting pair of trousers.

Shop Your Options

Realizing there are different shopping experiences can help take the dread out of shopping or help you when you don't enjoy a particular kind of shopping.

For instance, maybe you like to shop, but it's for household items or decorating stuff. And the thought of having to find some tops to fill a hole in your wardrobe feels more like a chore. Maybe you feel so overwhelmed with an ongoing work project or home renovation, you don't know how you'll find the time to get some new trousers to accommodate those extra few pounds you put on after the baby. Remember, you don't have to spend the day at the mall and

shop til you drop! There are many easy ways to tackle shopping and five of the easiest are:

    1. Window Shopping. Yes, this is still shopping!

    2. Hit the Stores

    3. Shop Online

    4. Shop Catalogues

    5. Hire me!

Check it out... Try it On... or Send it Home!

1. **Window Shopping** – This has great value. Taking the time
to walk around and check out what's currently in the stores
can actually teach you a lot. You'll see what's "in" you'll get
some inspiration, and the pressure's off if you know you
don't have to buy it yet. Also, when you actually "shop-shop"
you're in what I call the "me mindset." Meaning you are looking for things that would work for you, but you let all your
old habits and idiosyncrasies get in the way. But if you're just
strolling around enjoying the time out, you sort of take yourself out of your way. Instead of being bogged down by "I

can never get away with…" and "I can't wear that because…" you just take it in.

Also, since the goal of window shopping is learning and not buying, you can go into stores you wouldn't ordinarily frequent. And you can really have fun going to all the places that are usually out of your budget! Have a good time with it. Touch the fabrics, learn from the details of well made and high quality clothing. This will help you be a better judge of the quality and details of the items that are more budget friendly when you do go out to buy. You can also discover some wonderful sales racks at these chic places or put something on your wish list that be purchased later with a bonus check, some birthday money, or other windfall.

2. **Hit the Stores** – This of course is the most traditional way to shop. It's what you're used to. One of the questions I get asked a lot is "Where do I go to shop?" My advice is, before you decide what stores to go to, decide how you would like to shop. And give some thought to what's important to you. Is it price? Finding what you need easily? One-stop shopping? What would be the best way for you to stay inspired while you shop?

For example:

If you are easily overwhelmed in big stores, then your local TJ Maxx will frustrate you. A small boutique with very helpful sales people might be more to your liking.

If you aren't a people person and get irritated the first time someone asks if they can help you, then an intimate little shop is going to get on your nerves.

If you love the hunt, a few discount stores will garner you some great bargains – with a little work and patience.

If you are a kamakazi "buyer" and not a "shopper" then you need a place where you either know where everything is or where the staff is so trained, you can just describe what you need and let them do the scurrying.

If you only have an hour and your list is long, a big department store might be just the ticket. Another thing to consider is the time of day you'll be shopping. If you hate crowds, then early afternoon on tax free Saturday isn't the thing. If you only have half an hour to shop, then be smart – take that time to peruse the store, get your bearings, see if you like what you see and then be willing to come back later.

3. **Shop Online** – What an easy and "safe" way to shop! The huge surge in online shopping shows that many people agree with that. The convenience of online shopping is apparent. Anything you want or need is delivered straight to your door – it's like wardrobe takeout! Timing is a great advantage here, too. Shopping does take time and when you're smart shopping, then often "slow and steady wins the race" is a good

adage. So if your time is limited, shopping online at your convenience when you have the time to sit in front of the computer can really take the pressure off. And if you've been window shopping, you might have a great idea of what you're looking for.

There are some disadvantages of course. You obviously can't try things on and with the importance of fit, it's a challenge figuring out how to buy clothes that will look good on you from the computer screen. But there are ways to deal with this. Some online shops will offer free return shipping. Some even offer free shipping both ways.

There are also stores like J.Crew that allow you to buy things online and return them to the store. So even if the fit doesn't work, you're not stuck with anything. Also, as you get more practice at buying fits and sizes right for you, getting specific silhouettes that are flattering for your body type, and when you get familiar with the sizes of certain online sites, you'll get better at ordering.

A good experiment when you want to try more online shopping is to try stuff on in the physical stores of the online sites when they have one and make a note of their sizes that are right for you. Then you'll know what to get. Also, many online retailers offer reviews of items. Feedback from other buyers is a great way to determine how something will fit.

4. **Shop with Catalogues** – There's pretty much a catalogue for almost everything! Back in the late 1800's and early 1900's, you could even order your HOUSE through a catalogue. So you can certainly find a good catalogue or two for your ward-

robe needs! A catalogue doesn't wear your eyes out, lets you see items clearly, and often has really great extra information about the item, their sizes, etc. Their return policies are similar to online stores, with some free returns, postage stickers, packaging, etc, usually included in your order in case you need to send something back.

Once you order a few times, you'll find that you begin receiving more catalogues that are similar to what you've already bought from. Rather than be annoyed by that, just keep an open mind and a stack handy for when you're just sitting in the yard on a gorgeous evening or sipping a glass of wine or cup of tea in your down time. Just be sure to recycle them!

5. **Hire a Personal Stylist** – In my opinion (and this is what I do for my own clients), a good personal stylist will teach you how to be a smart shopper, find new styles you would have never tried, and show you easy ways to get the most use out of what you buy. It's amazing the confidence you can gain with a little shopping help. The knowledge you gain is priceless because you use it over and over again. (For specific information on how to work with me be sure to check out my website at

stylewithlee.com. It doesn't matter where you live – I can help!)

No matter how or where you buy it, there are easy questions you can ask yourself about any potential purchase:

1. Does it reflect the style I want to portray?

2. Does it fit properly? (And if not, am I willing to have it tailored?)

3. Am I willing to take care of it as the label directs?

4. Does it go with at least two other outfits?

5. Do I LOVE it?

Spend / Thrift

A big part of being disciplined when shopping is not over-spending. It's very easy to let that happen. But a great way to make shopping a better experience is to take away the guilt of spending too much money. Sticking to a budget is a snap with some simple tools.

• Bring cash – Duh, right? Just bring along the amount you want to spend in cash. When the cash runs out, you can quit while you're ahead. This also helps you avoid impulse decisions. When you think about those bills disappearing from your wallet, it might make you think twice if you're not totally in love with something you want to bring home from the store.

• Bring a list – You know how it is when you don't bring a list to the grocery store or Wal Mart or Target, right? Well, this is doubly true when you're clothes shopping. This also helps when you're trying to avoid impulse purchases.

• Put it on hold – If you are still thinking of an item 24 hours later, that's a sign of a potentially smart purchase. This eliminates impulse buying and buyer's remorse.

• Phone a friend – If you're on the urge of a splurge, phone a friend to purge that urge! Now of course I'm joking but it's a great way to avoid doing many silly things, not the least of which is to buy something you really don't need. But make sure you don't call your shopaholic pal!

• This sounds odd. But go ahead and splurge every once and a while – don't suck the fun out of shopping. If you can afford it, that is. If you're strapped right now or go overboard, then all the fun of a splurge is lost in feeling guilty the next day.

• Know how much you're earning and spending – Remember, each dollar represents a portion of your life – you traded your time and energy for it. Where is it going? Are you really getting fulfillment for each dollar spent on those new clothes?

Small Change

Now, talking about budgets and discipline isn't meant to be a killjoy. Let's talk about some other ways to have more fun shopping.

• Don't get stuck in a store rut! Does your car automatically drive to only two or three stores? Do you only go to discount stores and never go high faluting with the local swank shop?

~ It's not that finding a place where you feel comfortable and secure isn't great. But you might be surprised at how much more stimulating it is to branch out a little.

~ If you go to a certain store, it's likely it has a certain style. The problem with this is that even stores can get in a rut. If a store tends to turn out reincarnates of what you already have and you're not a disciplined shopper, you may find that you end up with a boring wardrobe that may scream that store's name, but not your style.

• Change up what you buy, too. Being original, trying something new, even choosing the unexpected is a great way to make yourself feel chic and modern. And it reminds you to have fun and not take style too seriously. Maybe it'll be a hit and you'll have another new element of "you."

~ Being in a fashion rut can make you dated.

~ If you always have a go-to look, you're going to come across as a rerun!

~ Bad habits are seldom attractive – are your clothes or shopping excursions a bad habit?

~ Always buying or wearing the same colors or patterns makes you a repeat offender!

I can't tell you how many times I see tons of black and white patterned shirts hanging in the same closet! Just take a close look at what's in your arms before going into that changing room. Just because it's a different pattern than the four you have hanging in your closet doesn't mean it's not the same note you've been playing in your style song.

CPW Formula

A great tool to determine whether or not a piece of clothing is a good deal or a good investment is to calculate it's CPW, or its Cost-Per-Wear. This is when your calculator comes in handy.

The cost per wear (CPW) is the price of an item divided by how many times you think you can wear it.

Let's say you have a new coat on your style / buy list. You

find a great looking trench coat that you love and are contemplating whether or not it is a good deal. The coat is on sale for $400. It is classic and neutral. You live in a chilly climate and even the summer has cool evenings. When you think about it, you think you could probably wear it once a week for most of the year? Well, that computes to the following:

52 weeks in a year, estimating wearing the coat once per week.

$400 divided by 52 = $7.69 per wear.

Pretty awesome deal.

Now let's say that you also found a funky jacket you adore – it's on sale and it's cheaper at $100. It's very trendy – it's what's hot right now. But it's way heavier and more colorful. It's not as transferable from season to season as the trench would be. But you could easily wear it a few times this season for sure.

3 times is a reasonable guess for how much you'd wear it this year.

$100 divided by 3 = $33.33 per wear.

Not as good of a deal!

Which is the better investment? If you said the trench, you're right! Knowing the CPW formula is a great tool to have when you're trying to decide whether or not to buy something. It adds a dose of reality to your shopping decisions and ensures you make decisions based on what works for your style, and not an emotional pull.

After-Stock

Hopefully once you've come home from the stores, you won't go into aftershock. But you can "After Stock" which is just a silly way of taking stock of what you've bought and what you're doing in general. Not all shopping savvy practices are done at the store. Here are some great tips that can help you be a smart shopper even after the stuff has come home from the store.

> 1. Try on everything you buy – AGAIN. Make sure you can still answer yes to all of your shopping guidelines once you are at home. If you bought shoes, give them a practice run. Wear them around the house to make sure they are really as comfortable as they were in the store. Put on that new blouse and make sure the snug sleeves are comfortable in all positions. Sit up and down and just sit in your new trousers or bottoms. Sometimes a bad crotch fit isn't apparent until you quit standing up! Yeeow!

2. Save and keep your receipts in one place. This way, if you need to return something, you can get a full refund and not have to just exchange. Just as a precaution, leave the tags on until you actually wear something out of the house.

3. Create a "New Items" section in your closet. As you wear each new item, integrate it into the proper wardrobe section of the closet.

4. Assess your new items section of the closet at least every month. If an item is still in the new section after that much time, you might want to just take it back for a refund or a more useful item. (Check your receipts right away. Some full refunds only apply within 30 days of the purchase. You'd hate to waste a refund just because you neglected to check your new stuff in a timely fashion.)

5. Schedule a time to play dress up in your closet! Come up with outfits that incorporate pieces you've just bought. Take pictures of outfits you create to reference on those days when you need inspiration but lack dressing brain power. Make notes about any new holes you see that need filling.

SHOP SHEET

Make copies of this sheet to take with you when you go shopping to help you stay on track and have a style you love.

Goals:

I am only looking for clothes that make me look and feel:

Items to add versatility / fill a hole / meet a current need are:

By budget is: $_____

Ready, Set, Shop

Shopping preparation Checklist:

_____ I know what's in my closet and what I need.

_____I am wearing clothes and shoes that are easy to remove and comfy.

_____I am clear on my style goals.

_____I have brought wardrobe pieces that I want to make additional outfits with.

_____I am wearing the proper undergarments.

Chapter 10
Keep it Up!

Seldom do people discern eloquence under a threadbare
cloak.
—Juvenal

Hopefully after doing your style homework here, a good
closet edit, and learning to shop like a pro, you are feeling
inspired to see that dressing really is an art. Just like I said in
the beginning, choosing an outfit helps you paint a picture
and your picture tells the story of you! Let's revisit some of
the tips I gave you earlier.

Have you come up with some new outfits using what
you already have in your closet – hopefully by repurposing some items from one segment and putting
them with items from another segment?

Have you come up with some new outfits incorpo-
rating anything new you might have acquired with
something you already had?

Have you experimented a little by trying something
you wouldn't ordinarily use? Like a color you think
you should wear, an accessory that's a bit unexpected,
or a couple of "neutrals" paired with something you
wouldn't ordinarily pair them with?

Trend Blend

Trends get a bad rap. That's because so many people blindly follow them, looking like the latest issue of "Can't Think for Myself Magazine" or because a runway trend is taken too literally. Many people think that only the young can wear current trends and so they avoid looking up to date in a misguided attempt to be "timeless." But timeless doesn't mean not current. There are many ways to infuse a current trend into your wardrobe without veering away from your style goals and without looking like you're trying too hard.

Silhouettes

Trends are fun and you should have fun dressing at any age. A great tip for infusing a trend into your wardrobe is to stick with the silhouettes and shapes that already look great on you. In a trend cycle, silhouettes change the slowest. Much slower than color, print, fabric, embellishment, etc. So if a certain trend is everywhere, see if you can find that print, fabric, or whatever in your tried and true silhouettes.

Good is in the Details

A great way to incorporate a trend into your wardrobe is in the details of an outfit. Stitching, buttons, cuffs, piping, draping, texture… all these are super easy to add to your closet without breaking the bank and without being a slave to fashion.

Bend the Trend

If your first impulse about a seasonal trend is it's not for you, just have an open mind and think outside the box. Maybe snakeskin is all the rage – if you can't bear to have a motley-print around your waist or on your feet, maybe you can find a belt, shoes, or purse with a snakeskin texture but in a solid, neutral, or unexpectedly bright color. If fur is everywhere and even the ethical choice of faux fur intimidates you, maybe there's a cute little clutch out there, or a chic jacket with just a touch of fur on the collar. It's not that you must incorporate every trend. It's just that trends are a great and easy way to keep feeling fresh and add those little tweaks that keep your style looking current.

Accessory Necessity

While there are certain accessories that are timeless, you'll
find that they can be used in new ways to reflect updates.
A lovely, heirloom gemstone pin can go from "churchy"
or "granny" to funky just by pinning it to your artsy, hand
knitted cap or putting it on a long, slim piece of leather as a
necklace.

And of course, accessories are often the easiest way
to incorporate a new look. A wild print, funky color, even
elements like fringe or feathers or whatever is current is much
easier to pull off in a belt, purse, shoes, or jewelry.

Time Warp

Does everyone you haven't seen in a while say the same thing,
"You haven't changed a bit!" Well, you might want to take
a look at what that means. Hopefully it means that you're
face is fresh, your hair looks great, and you have a marvelous
bounce in your step. But it's time to ask yourself an honest
question if you get that a lot – or even if you don't. "Do I
look, dress, style myself, and / or have the same hair as I did
as a young 'un?

You may be rockin' those 80's bangs, you may be
skinny enough to fit into that 90's style "skort" and you may
still have groovy, long hippy hair. But it might be time for an

update. Don't worry, this doesn't mean you have to lose your signature look. It just means you can incorporate it and update it into your style. Rather than look like a cliché', can you find a way to take an element from your glory days and add it to your wardrobe (rather than letting it dominate it)? A cool hemp bracelet might be just the element of surprise you need for that chic, sexy, jersey knit dress. Maybe a structured denim skirt that's a bit longer could be an updated version of your famous mini or skort. Or maybe some vintage glasses can add the touch of geek you like.

Prioritize

One thing you must remember, always, is to keep making yourself a priority! Look, I know how it is – this is my whole business, and yet I'm still constantly amazed at how easy it is to fall off my own priority list! It's really easy when you're juggling many things to put yourself, and your style, last. But don't do that. The farther you fall or the longer you're not even on your own priority list, you may get into bad thought habits.

Don't look in the mirror and wonder where the girl of your past went. Don't feel self conscious because of that extra weight or those new lines on your face. Remember what you learned in the beginning of this book – style isn't about being self-obsessed or vain. It's about expression and who you are on the inside.

* If you've already fallen off your priority list don't despair. Style is often times the first thing you lose, but it's easy to get back. And you've already got the tools you need to make it happen.

Chapter 11
Travel with Style

One's destination is never a place, but a new way of seeing things.
—Henry Miller

Whether going by plains, trains, or automobiles, traveling – like dressing and shopping – can be an art. With the huge change in security measures in airports worldwide, it has become more imperative than ever to be a savvy packer and traveler. Packing for a variety of occasions, especially if you have many different types of things to do, can be stressful enough in and of itself – when you add the size, weight, and other restrictions of carry on luggage to the mix, a simple business trip or much needed getaway could turn into something that puts a damper on your travel-with-style excursion. I'm here to help you de-stress that packing process and feel great about your clothing options once you arrive at your destination, no matter how you get there.

Bag It!

Wouldn't it be great if it were the old days – when you could pack your steamer trunks and have all your things brought straight to your room with the clothes already hanging in their mini closet and even have all your little crystal vials filled up in their cubbies with your necessities in them? Well, those days are over – but you can sometimes feel like you're lugging a big old trunk around if you have the wrong travel equipment.

Before we even get into planning your travel wardrobe, packing, and traveling, let's start with your bag. You need to carefully consider what kind of bag you buy or travel with.

> **For example:** A soft, wonderfully patterned bag (like Vera Bradley and the like) is almost miraculously roomy, comfy to carry, and looks adorable. But it's not made to handle being man handled, it's lack of structure will wrinkle everything you bring, and it would be easy to get into if someone were so inclined. Save these bags for short car trips and to carry around on a more daily basis if you need to tote a lot of stuff around with you.

> A crazy-expensive designer luggage set may scream fashion and style, but it may also holler "really expensive stuff in here!" You can pay more for luggage than you do for your trip! And if something happens to ruin it, you'll be sick with guilt over the investment.

> A bag with tons of bells and whistles might be more hassle than helpful. A bunch of zippers and snaps and buckles will greatly add to the weight of it. And while pockets are handy, if there are too many, you'll spend all your time hunting for stuff.

The fabric of the bag should be durable and not inclined to pick up every speck of dirt it encounters. Light colored bags of course will get dingy if great care isn't taken.

Try out the strap in the store. Does it rub you? Is it really stiff and unwieldy? Are there alternative straps with it if you want to change the length of them?

If your bag has wheels, check them out. Are they so cheap they'll get busted up or fall off? Are they of good quality? How do they roll? Don't depend on a brand – really check this stuff out.

The more structured the bag, and the harder the sides, the more control you have over how things travel inside. A very firm, hard sided bag is also quite roomy inside even if it's diminutive. (There's a reason pilots and flight attendants carry those types of bags!)

If you're doing most of your traveling on the road, a hard, unyielding suitcase might be harder to handle, especially if others are traveling with you. Something with more of a squish might be handier.

A very unique color or pattern might make your bag instantly recognizable on the luggage claim conveyor belt. But are you still going to be in love with a purple plaid suitcase in the long run? Choose the look wisely.

And of course, once you have the bag, put your information on it immediately in case it becomes lost. You should do this even is you are not flying. You just never know. Put your initials on it and just a phone number – you don't need to give all of your information out to a potential stalker or thief. If you're flying, put a little something on your bag that's easily recognizable when it's gliding past with dozens of other bags. I use a bright, fluorescent, reflective little piece of tape on my bag handle, or a bright and interesting bag tag.

Back to the Basics

The key to looking and feeling stylish when you travel is to bring clothing that can be mixed and matched to create different outfits. This means you have to pack with outfits in mind. You can't just grab bottoms you love and tops you love, dresses you love, and all your favorite pieces. They might be your faves but that doesn't mean it's all going to automatically go together. And you're certainly a captive audience when you get there. Not that folks don't often love shopping in a new place – but if you're limited in time, in budget, or otherwise not inclined to feel the push of buying an outfit for something important because the stuff you brought with you doesn't work, then this first step is crucial.

This is a great time to go back through the section about foundational planning and color. When you're putting together some things for your journey, you'll want to remember the tips on neutrals (and their clever pairing with unexpected items), pseudo neutrals, etc. Making outfits with neutrals or pseudo neutrals when you travel can help you pair down the number of clothes you need to bring.

And don't forget the lesson on the equation for the perfect outfit you learned earlier – even neutrals can be put together in such a way as to create a great outfit.

Key item + Supporting Item + Completer Piece + Pizzazz = A perfect showcase for your style!

Less is More

The way to carry less stuff with you is to think of one word: VERSATILITY. Don't get caught up in fearing that you may need this and may need that and keep adding to your luggage. Stick to these tips and you'll find it all a snap.

• Pick a color palette – If you just had a flashback to the simpler life when you were a kid and wish Garanimals came in adult sizes, that's exactly what I mean. Choose a palette that works with one color of shoe and can be mixed and matched with many other items you plan to pack.

• Choose key pieces in neutral colors – Decide on what key pieces you need. A suit? Black pants? Skirts? Jeans? Shorts?

• Also choose key pieces that you can dress up or down – like a wrap dress.

• Use completer pieces to layer with during travel. It is always both hot and cold when you travel, whether you're riding in a car or flying. Completer pieces like jackets, cardigans, or scarves can be used to jazz up your outfits and keep you warm.

• Make sure everything can serve double duty. This means your scarf can be used as a shawl for warmth or as an accessory to your outfit. Or a striped top can go with a pair of trousers, under a blazer, or with some cute shorts. Or a pair of stretchy pants that can serve as PJ's for a night before becoming your work out pants the next morning. Each item that can do double duty helps you save a spot in your suitcase.

• Neutral or pseudo neutral *accessories* will be just as handy as neutral or pseudo neutral key *items*! A camel purse and gold clutch can go from day to evening for an entire week, for example.

My favorite traveling pseudo neutral is a red shoe. It goes with everything and has pizzazz at the same time!

Location, Location, Location

These seem like rather obvious questions, but if you take a moment to think about them before packing, you can do some planning that will make the packing easier. Why don't you jot some notes down about the following?

1. Where are you going? Not just generally, but specifically, like will you be staying at a hotel that has hair dryers and irons or at a friend's house where you will need to watch what you wear to bed? Will you be going to several places? Will you have to walk everywhere or are taxis or car rentals available?

2. What will the weather likely be like? Are you from a warm climate traveling to a cold climate? Layers can help keep you from sweating on the way to and from your car at the airport as you can quickly slip them off. Are you going to a place famous for rain? A trench coat takes up way more room than an umbrella.

3. How long will you be gone? If you're going for an extended period but won't be seeing the same people all the time, is there a way to do laundry? That way you could pack half as much. Is it a super short business trip where you practically have to go straight from the airport to a taxi to a board meeting?

4. What will you be doing? You need a clear idea of your daily agenda. Does the boss love to insist the whole team go golfing when out of town together? Will you have to schmooze with a client at a swank restaurant?

5. Who are you going with? Your family could care less if you wear something multiple times, but girls-on-the-town means dressing up for fun. If you're with business colleagues you must remember that even on your off hours your still at work. Professional attire is a must.

On the next page is an example of a handy travel chart to give you an idea of what we just went over. This is a chart I made for myself.

Travel Day	Function/ Activity	Day	Evening	Accessories	Extras
Monday	Travel, dinner with colleagues	Trouser Jean, grey suit jacket, white T shirt	Wrap dress	Day: Bold necklace, metallic wedge flat Night: Bold neck-lace, red heel, metal-lic clutch	Pashmina for chic layering on plane (or folded up for a pillow)
Tuesday	Meetings, casual dinner with colleagues	Grey pantsuit, patterned blouse	Patterned blouse, trouser jean	Day: black pump, simple jewelry Night: me-tallic flat, pashmina	Leather portfolio, professional computer bag
Wednesday	Meetings, dressy dinner with colleagues	Wrap dress, grey suit jacket	Little black dress	Day: black pump, bold necklace Night: bold necklace, red heel, pashmina	Patterned or chic hosiery, brooch for jacket lapel
Thursday	Breakfast with boss, travel home	Grey suit trousers, white T shirt, burgundy cardigan		Metallic flat, brooch	Belt for cardigan

So after filling this out, my packing list is:

Clothes

Grey Suit

2 white T shirts

Trouser jean

Cardigan

Wrap dress

Little black dress

Accessories

Pashmina

Brooch

Bold necklace

3 pairs of shoes (metallic flats, red heels, black pumps)

Hosiery

Copy and enlarge the chart on the next page, print a copy from my blog (stylewithlee.com/blog), or make one up yourself to make packing for your next trip simply effortless!

Packing Chart

Travel Day	Function/ Activity	Day	Evening	Accessories	Extras
Monday					
Tuesday					
Wednesday					
Thursday					
Friday					
Saturday					
Sunday					

The most versatile items for any trip include:

Bold necklace

Scarf / Pashmina

Metallic clutch

Nude shoe

Pseudo neutral day bag (You can use it as a sly carry on when flying!)

Here's a bonus checklist. Make a copy of this to check off
when you are getting everything together and as a final step
to know you haven't forgotten anything.

CLOTHES

_____Day outfits

_____Evening outfits

_____Excursion / Activity outfits

_____Layering pieces for travel (cardigans, jackets, etc.)

_____Coat

_____Gym clothes

_____Bathing suit

_____Undergarments (proper type and color)

_____Socks /Hosiery

_____Pajamas

_____Shoes

_____Scarf / Wrap

_____Day bag

_____Evening bag

_____Collapsible tote bag

TOILETRIES

_____Hair products and tools

_____Skincare products

_____Sunscreen

_____Dental hygiene products

_____Razor / Shaving cream

_____Deodorant

_____Eye care (contact solution, eyeglasses and case..)

_____Make up

_____Feminine supplies

_____First aid (aspirins or ibuprophen, etc. sinus medication, prescriptions, band aids, etc.)

_____Insect repellent (if you're outdoors)

MUST-HAVES

_____Travel entertainment (books, magazines, ipod, etc.)

_____Charged mobile phone and charger

_____Proper Identification

_____$$$ (Cash and credit cards, money orders if needed, etc.)

_____Tickets

_____Itinerary

_____Destination phone numbers and addresses, and / or directions (make a copy for loved ones at home)

_____Sunglasses

_____Compact mirror

_____Touch up make up (for your purse)

_____Camera and camera accessories

_____Plastic bags (like ziplocs – you'd be surprised how much you use them)

_____Lock for baggage

_____Notebook / pens

_____Binoculars (little mini ones are really invaluable)

_____*For overseas travel, Electrical converter & plug adapter

_____Flashlight and batteries (if you're doing outdoorsy things)

Fly By

I get asked for insider travel tips a lot. Now that I've got you ready to pack like a pro, here are a few tips about making travel (especially air travel) easy.

To Wear En Route

1. What is comfy but not slobby. Skip the sweats or yoga pants. Choose trousers or jeans with a little stretch in the fabric.

2. What you feel good in. It never fails, dress like a slob and you'll meet someone well-heeled and fascinating. Remember that airports and planes are great people watching places – make sure you're worth watching! – and they are great places to chat with new and interesting people. Dress as if you expect to meet someone exciting on your journey – who knows, maybe you will.

3. Layers. I've said it before but it bears repeating. There's nothing worse than being too hot or too cold when you're traveling. Planes are usually hot during taxiing and cold during flight. Even when you're riding in the car, sometimes your companion likes things cooler or warmer than you.

4. Your bulkiest items when flying. This sounds weird but I think it works.

> A coat – It saves tons of room in your suitcase, not to mention its weight, and a jacket can even act as a carry on as you can store things in its pockets and a blanket if you get cold on the flight. It's easily stored in the overhead if you need to.

> Shoes – If you're bringing bulky shoes, can you wear them instead of pack them? Personally, I'm not bothered by taking off my shoes at security (you usually only have to go through it one time) and with a little prep work you can do it quickly and efficiently without too much bother.

Pack wrinkle free fabrics like cashmere, silks, and rayons. Some travel sites that carry good travel clothes (but you have to be selective so you don't end up looking frumpy) are travelsmith.com and magellans.com.

A trick when you are packing to eliminate wrinkles is to place tissue paper in between your clothes. When they are folded, they slide around on the tissue instead of settling into each other – causing wrinkles.

I'm also a fan of the rolling method of packing, which I think saves the most room and helps keep things relatively wrinkle free.

Shoe Fly

When you are traveling, it's best to limit your shoes. Here are some ways to bring shoes with you without unnecessary hassle.

1. Like I mentioned before, wear the bulkiest ones. If you must pack them, utilize their interior for packing space by bagging socks or small accessories and slipping them in.

2. Bag your shoes separately in order to strategically fit them into the puzzle that is your suitcase. This also prevents your clothes from getting dirty or smelling like shoes.

3. If you have a soft travel bag, use shoes on the bottom or on the sides to reinforce your bag.

Ditty Bag

Check out the place you're staying. It's not just the swank places that offer complimentary toiletries. There might also be a store there where you can purchase some of these items – because toiletries take up an awful lot of space in your luggage. Also, some items can do double duty. You can use conditioner on your legs instead of packing bulky shaving cream. If you're not into makeup, perhaps a tinted moisturizer with sunscreen will do nicely for both.

- Ditch your special toiletry bag if you are short on luggage space – although nice to bring into the bathroom with you, it takes up tons of space. Try using ziplock bags instead.

- Get rid of all unnecessary packaging to pair down.

- Get your own small containers or go to the travel section of the drugstore for minis.

- Be sure to check out the latest regulations regarding liquids on the airline you're traveling on.

Last Blast

I know I've given you tons of tips. But here are some further ideas that may really help you get there with a smile.

Wear your heaviest items.

Don't overstuff your bags.

Unpack as SOON as you reach your destination.

Sometimes shipping can be more cost effective – check it out.

Your heaviest items should be on the bottom of your suitcase.

Pack more tops than bottoms. (Bottoms take up more room, are heavier, and can be easily worn more than once.)

Wear or keep with you the most important belongings.

For some insider tips on specific vacation and packing challenges (think African safaris, international destinations, cruises and the like), please reference my blog stylewithlee. com/blog. Another great spot is onebag.com!

44 lbs / 20 kkgs is the weight restriction for international flights. But you are allowed 2 bags. Be sure to research the country you're going to, and the regions within that country, for exceptions. Also check out the airlines you are traveling on. You might find that international flights to that country allows the above weight, for example, but when you try to travel to certain regions you can only take much less weight in your luggage. Airlines vary in what they allow and what you're allowed to bring. Do your homework so you can enjoy your trip.

Chapter 12
The Business of Style

We are all in the business of getting dressed.
—Nina Garcia

When career opportunities knock, does your image and style answer? And let's be frank. When your style answers, is it ultimately helping you to make money? Style is personal, yes. And it's a reflection of your true self, yes. But you can leverage your style to help you achieve the business success you deserve.

> *Disclaimer* – This isn't about putting on an outfit just to pretend you are someone you are not in order to get business. What I mean by leveraging your image is simply polishing your style and ensuring that you shine so that more clients or opportunities come your way. A great connection you meet at a networking event, an exciting new customer, or even a conversation in line at the grocery store can lead to a totally unexpected opportunity. Make sure you're dressed for it!

Your image is actually a sales tool – it is the strongest marketing tool you have and it is one that you have complete control over. Think of it this way: If you pay to advertise in a magazine and they print your phone number incorrectly, you can't do a lot to fix it until the next printing – IF you decide to give your ad rep another chance that is. But you can fix a style challenge anytime (or avoid it altogether) by what you choose to wear each day when you walk out the door.

If you think I'm exaggerating, think of it this way. Have you ever picked out produce in a grocery store? If you're picking out a lovely tomato for dinner, how many do you have to look at before choosing the perfect one? What about the super wonderful ones at the farmer's market or the organic food store? It's hard to figure out which one is the best choice.

On the other side of the spectrum, if you see a hundred gorgeous bananas stacked up and one is bruised and not-so-fresh looking, would you buy that one? Or how about cereal? Would you grab the box that is slightly crushed? If you were looking at the canned goods, would you choose a can that was dented? Or had a torn, sloppy looking label? If image affects the way you buy a simple ingredient for a single meal, imagine how it can affect whether or not customers choose to do business with you!

1st Place

Let's talk about first impressions. I mentioned the old phrase before, "You never get a second chance to make a first impression." It's true. Studies show it takes only seven seconds to make a first impression! Let that sink in. You have seven seconds to say who you are! Because of those seven seconds, whoever sees you who is in a position to affect your business has jumped to conclusions about who you are, whether or not they want to work with you or your company, or even how much you can be paid or if you can be trusted.

When in doubt about what to wear for a first meeting (and impression) with someone you have no knowledge about, remember that it is better to be over dressed than under dressed. You can always remove your jacket for a more casual look once you arrive.

If you're still not sold on putting value in first impressions, here are some statistics from a study done by a sociolinguist by the name of Albert Merabian.

In a face-to-face encounter – whether at a networking event, an interview, or a dinner party…

-7% of others' judgment comes from the words you use.

-38% comes from the vocal tone and inflection you use.

-55% of the message transmitted comes from your appearance.

Just like any style issue, this isn't about ego – in the current competitive business environment, a polished appearance is considered a basic job requirement. Let me elaborate on that. Your image is basically made up of your wardrobe, your grooming habits, and your non verbal communication. Combined, these factors frame you as competent, knowledgeable, employable, powerful, and / or anything else you choose to communicate. And don't forget my wardrobe rule – let your clothes do lots of the work for you.

If your pitch to a client includes how well your company delivers on time, then you better be on time to your meetings. Or if you believe (or claim) you beat out the competition because you are so attentive to every single detail a customer needs, your appearance has to back that up. Scuffed shoes or a poor fitting suit doesn't scream detail oriented.

But I don't want to stress you out. In fact, there's reason to be thrilled that how you are styled makes such a big difference. Todd Lyon, author of *Mastering the New ABC's of What to Wear to Work,* says, "Clothing is both a powerful communicator and an important business tool. Though judgment via fashion might seem unfair, in fact it presents a wonderful opportunity. By dressing to reflect your career objectives, you can send potent messages about your team spirit, ambition, creativity, and professionalism."

Isn't that wonderful? What a fabulous way to think about your style. Basically, you can draw a picture of how you see yourself as a business person – and an asset to those you want to do business with – and then dress yourself in order to present that idea. You can be responsible, detail oriented, timely, relevant, bold, even cutting edge – all in one outfit.

Again, it's about letting your style do a lot of the work for you, not stressing about how important how you dress is.

Think of it this way. How much would you pay someone to magically influence a client to be inclined toward giving you what you want? Well, that first seven-second impression does just that.

Proof Reader

The great thing is, you can apply all the same practices you already use in order to be a smart business person to your business style with wonderful results. If this sounds like too much work, just consider the amount of time and energy you put into writing something as simple as an email to someone important, much less something like a proposal or a bid. If it's someone you need to make a good impression on, then you better believe you will proof that communiqué before letting the person in question read it.

Yep, you guessed it. It's time to think about proofing your wardrobe. Let me ask you a question:

If every day you knew you would have the opportunity to go after your biggest client yet, what would you want to be wearing?

I believe that's a great way to think about putting your work wardrobe together. Because you never know when the great opportunities will come.

Brand News

Business women are constantly thinking about marketing. Let's think about your image from a marketing perspective. Think about a company like Apple. Their commercials, their packaging, the experience you have in their stores... all make you think of a cutting edge, hip, and fun brand. They've done such a good job branding themselves that just seeing their apple logo makes you feel cutting edge, hip, and fun. When you purchase their product, it's like you're in the club – the cool girl. All because of an apple!

Your clothes can do the same thing for you. Your entire appearance tells people your message, or the three words you came up with earlier. Your clothes help to reinforce this message.

The Three Key

Remember how helpful it was when you wrote down words to describe yourself early in the book? Take a moment to think how those words translate in your professional world.

In my case, three of the words I chose were sexy, approach-able, and unique. So choosing clothing that has that particular feel makes me feel confident, at work as well as at play. That doesn't mean I plan on wearing a low cut blouse or a short skirt to work. No way! I channel sexy into my professional wardrobe by choosing a structured dress that fits well. When clothing fits, I feel sexy, and therefore am confident to do my job well

I recently worked with a virtual client who had chosen the word "rocker" as one of her three key words. She auto-matically assumed that she had to leave her "rocker side" at home. Quite the contrary! I asked her a few questions about what felt "rocker" to her. One thing she mentioned was wear-ing leather. Obviously she couldn't come to work in a short leather mini-skirt – but why not wear a fabulous leather blazer with a pencil skirt or trouser? The leather was a nod to her inner rocker chic, but the type of leather jacket kept her look professional.

So why don't you take a moment and think about how your three key words can be translated for your work? Don't forget to post your words somewhere in your closet. Before you walk out the door, ask yourself if your clothing is really sending the message you want.

It's a Tie

Ah, details. Here's an interesting side note about our current

President, Barrack Obama. Believe it or not, since he took office there has been a lot of talk about when he wears a red tie versus a blue one. It seems he's breaking the mold of red as the only power tie color as a way of sending a message that he is one with the people – a regular guy. Red symbolizes confidence, action, royalty, and most is associated with power. Blue symbolizes trust, dependability, and peace. Whether you like President Obama or not, next time you see him on TV, I bet you'll notice his tie and give some thought to what message he is trying to send with his image during his speech.

It seems a minute detail, but it's obviously being noticed on our nation's leader. And it's a detail that men have to use to speak about who they are. Women have a much greater opportunity in that we have lots at our disposal to wow our colleagues and clients. We should take advantage of it!

Curb Appeal

Now that you've gotten a little more clarity on the message you want to send, you need to know how you can beat out your competition. I can tell you how in two fun words:

Curb appeal.

If you've ever bought or sold a house, you know all

about curb appeal. It's all your real estate agent talks about when listing your home, and it's what makes you want to stop and go in when you're driving by. Well, the way you dress is an easy way to give yourself curb appeal. When you stand up in a networking meeting, people will take notice. They mentally note the fact that they would like to meet you and learn more about what you do.

To add curb appeal to your image, I recommend dressing intentionally. Dressing intentionally is very different from dressing each morning just to put on clothes so you don't leave the house naked. When going to work, it is the process of thoughtfully putting together an outfit in order to achieve a goal.

No matter what, your wardrobe should always be:

1. **Appropriate**

2. **Professional**

3. **Comfortable**

4. **Strategic**

Take a long, hard look at your work style. Is it all of those things in addition to being an expression of you? Does your work wardrobe help you turn heads and profits? Let's look at these wardrobe ideas a little closer.

1. **Dressing Appropriately** – When your image is appropriate, you look like you belong in the industry in which you work in. That way you already look like an expert. We all want to be considered experts, right? And on the other side of that equation, when you hire someone or purchase a product, you want the best. If you don't look appropriate, people are going to doubt your qualifications and expertise.

> **For example:** Have you ever been to a networking meeting and someone in the IT field stands up and sells themselves as the company you need to stay updated on the cutting edge of technology... yet, this person looks frumpy and outdated – the exact opposite of cutting edge? Would you "buy" that person as someone that could get your business technology where it needed to go?

2. **Professional Dressing** – This seems like another no brainer. But it's amazing how easy it is to forget that your entire wardrobe must embody a professional feel. Dressing professionally means that you are dressed in a way that shows you are serious about what you do, and that you are good at it. Wearing business like clothing will give you confidence that you look the part, making you look and feel credible. Everything about your outfit must be professional. Details matter! And they will be noticed.

- Bag / Portfolio

- Overcoat

- Watch

- Shoes

3. **Dressing Comfortably** – A comfortable wardrobe means more than just clothes you feel comfortable in. You should be comfortable in three ways:

> First, you need to be comfortable with your body type and dress it in the most flattering way. Like I taught you before, this involves spending time learning about what your body really looks like, not what you think it looks like or wish it looks like. Correct fit can make you forget about your body insecurities, which in turn will make you feel happy, confident, and comfortable with yourself. This way you have one less thing to worry about when you're pitching to your ideal customer.

> Secondly, you should be comfortable expressing your personality, or personal style through your clothing. Your clothing should help send a message about who you are and why you or your company is the answer to your customer's need.

Lastly, your wardrobe does need to be physically comfortable. If you are uncomfortable in your clothes, you will shift and fidget, giving off nervous energy. If you have a new outfit you plan to wear to an important meeting or event, give it a trial run. Wear it around the house. Sit down. Stand up. Does everything stay in place? Are you wrinkled in minutes? Do you feel confident?

4. **Dressing Strategically** – This is one of the most important parts of dressing intentionally. It's something people often forget but it makes the most impact. If you want to succeed in your business, you must dress in a manner that shows you are the person / company for the job. Give some thought to your goals, your field, where you want your company to be in five years… This attention to detail often separates you from the rest of your colleagues and shows that you have what it takes to make your customers happy.

All this means you dress as if you are meeting with your biggest customers every day, even if there isn't a single meeting on the books – you never know when opportunity will knock. After all, you have to look the part before anyone is going to give it to you.

Each morning when you get dressed be as intentional as you are in other areas of your life. You wouldn't hire just anyone off the street. You wouldn't hire someone who was slovenly, or late to a first meeting with you. And you wouldn't be late for a meeting with a new client. Remember that example of choosing fruit – it's only human nature to be picky about what you want. Especially if it involves money!

Dynamic Duo

By dressing intentionally, you practice "duo-purpose" dressing. It makes you feel confident, which is the main purpose of clothing – besides just covering up nakedness. And here's an odd thing to think about regarding the importance of feeling good in your clothes: Americans have the opportunity to see their own reflection, in mirrors, windows, elevator doors, etc., up to 55 times a day!

That's 55 times to give yourself an extra little confidence boost. You walk past a mirror and think, "Okay, I'm ready. I look good!" (Which is certainly better than the alternative.) And having that attitude makes a potential customer feel confident in you.

Consistency

The final advice for leveraging your image to get the job success you want is to be consistent. In all areas of business, consistency is key. You go to Starbucks each morning because your coffee is consistently good. If you did not get consistently good coffee, what would you do? You'd stop going. The same applies to your work wardrobe, especially in order to use it as a leveraging tool. No matter where you are or what you are doing, your clothing is sending a message about you and your business.

Opportunity Knocks

One of the best things about business, no matter what type of business or industry you work in, is that opportunity is around every corner!

- Opportunity to interview for the perfect job.

- Opportunity to get your foot in the door at a prestigious firm.

- Opportunity for advancement.

- Or even opportunity for a complete and total career change.

Be dressed in your best when you step out of the door each morning!

Bonus Section: Interview with Style

Like you learned before, when your image is appropriate you look like you belong in the position, the company, and the industry you want. If you don't look appropriate, people are going to doubt your qualifications and expertise. Do your homework to learn what is appropriate for:

- The company you are interviewing with.

- The person who will be interviewing with.

How?

- Scour their website.

- Call HR and enquire about the dress code at the company.

- Sit in the parking lot and watch what people are wearing as they enter and exit.

> That might sound a bit stalkerish, but it is important you know what you're dealing with. It's hard enough to land a job these days – why wouldn't you gain every juicy bit of knowledge

you could to get ahead? Employers hire people they are confident will do a good job and fit in well with the existing company structure. Show them this is you by being appropriate – and looking like you'd be a perfect match for the team already in place.

Here's a scenario to get you thinking. This is totally stereotyping, but I'm just illustrating a point here:

Let's say you have interviews at two very different top public relations firms. What do you wear at each respective interview? After you've done your research, you determine that the 1st company sends a message that they are creative, fun, and refreshing. The 2nd company sends a message that they are traditional, powerful, and intelligent.

Company 1 interview outfit – Wear a suit that is a little more fun than traditional. Maybe a neutral suit like taupe or grey that has interesting detail to it, like a kick pleat in the skirt or with a bold pin stripe. Be a little more fun with a cool, closed toe platform heel. Maybe play with a pointy toe, a tassel, a tasteful adornment on the toe, etc.

Company 2 interview outfit – Wear a power suit in a neutral color like black, grey, or navy. Adding visual interest with a rich colored, collared shirt. Traditional, closed toe heel. Simple and tasteful jewelry.

Chapter 13
Clothes Minded

It has been my honor to guide you through this style journey. I really believe that taking the time for inner reflection, self-improvement, and education is so important. If only I would have learned that when I was in college! But it doesn't matter when you take the time to invest in yourself as long as you do it.

My good friend Jessica taught me a long time ago about having a PIP, a personal improvement plan. Your PIP doesn't have to be a massive undertaking, it can be as simple as learning a new recipe, treating yourself to coffee, or finding style you love. It's my hope that this book has shown you that great style really can be simple and effortless. Yes, it takes a little work up front but the payoff is huge. Once you know how to create style you love, it's a skill that stays with you. The knowledge is priceless.

This last, short chapter is a reminder that being clothes minded isn't about being egotistical. It's about being true to yourself! So give some thought to your own clothes. Do the items you own help you achieve the image you want? Hopefully if you've done the activities and learned the lessons from the previous chapters of this book, the answer is yes. If the items in your closet don't match your message, you may find that you wind up with a closet stuffed to the gills (even if it feels like you have nothing to wear). Why? Because there's a disconnect between what you have and buy and the way you want to be seen.

That's why the closet edit and the putting together of outfits and repurposing of items from different segments is so important. Not to mention filling in those wardrobe holes. But as you saw with these exercises and with all this great information, there's nothing to be stressed out about. In fact, there's reason to be thrilled that how you are styled makes such a big difference in your life!

Finding style you love gives you power. What you choose to wear is something you have complete control over. That is one of the coolest things about style. And that's not something you can say about many facets of life. Getting dressed is a decision. Each morning you can decide to wear clothing that makes you feel great or you can wear clothing that simply keeps you from being naked. Both take the same amount of time to put on, but having style you love affects you in amazing ways. It inspires you to do your best, it makes you a role model, and it makes you realize with the right knowledge anything is possible.

Your time for great style is NOW! If style is something that you've never really had, or have simply lost, I remind you that style is easy to find and simpler than you think to get back. Lucky you, you've got all the tools you need right here in this book. Take your time because worthwhile change doesn't happen overnight. You are on your way to Simply Effortless Style!

Here's to your style!

Meet Lee,
Your Style Expert

From 4H to Style Expert: My Story

My passion for helping people feel great about their style started at a young age when I became a proud member of the Stylish Stitchers, a local 4H club dedicated to teaching girls about sewing and design. I learned to make stylish wardrobe pieces and modeled them in 4H fashion shows.

My love for style continued into the fourth grade, when my best friend had to change schools, and we wanted to make sure she made a great first impression. It was at the age of eight that I found my calling as a style expert. I edited her closet, getting rid of all things childish and not fitting for a cool fourth grader. Together, we planned the outfits she would wear during her first week at a new school.

After college, I enjoyed a career as a retail merchandiser and sales representative for a large footwear and apparel company, but I always felt something was missing in my life.

It was not until my Dad promised to give my Mom $500 to go shopping if I would edit her closet that I realized I could help women everywhere achieve simple and effortless style. So, I quit my job, and in 2007, became a full-fledged style expert when I launched *Charleston Style Concierge*—which I rebranded as *Style with Lee* in 2012.

Style with Lee aims to show women that great style isn't about being egotistical; it's about achieving the confidence and happiness they deserve. The right clothes can make us feel invincible, giving us the confidence to accomplish anything we desire.

I am committed to helping women feel more confident through the development of personal style. I have worked with individual clients, helped corporations upgrade their employees' images, and spoken in front of groups teaching people how to achieve the style they want. No matter whom I'm working with, there is nothing more satisfying than watching my clients gain confidence with their new look. They stand taller, speak louder, and are proud of their new style knowledge.

As a College of Charleston graduate, I am passionate about giving back to my community. As a former partner of Charleston's chapter of Dress for Success, I promoted economic independence for disadvantaged women. While working with the group, I accepted donations from clients, organized fashion fundraising events, and sat on its Board of Directors.

In addition to my love for great style, I have always had a love for horses. An avid equestrian since age five, I spend my free time riding. I'm blessed to live in beautiful Charleston, South Carolina, with my husband, daughter, dog, and two cats.

For more information about me, check out the *Client Interview* on my website, stylewithlee.com. To book me for services or for an event, just click on the *services* tab on my homepage. I look forward to hearing from you.

Bonus: Resolve to Love Your Style!

You don't need a perfect body, tons of money, or an amazing fashion sense. All it takes is an adjustment of ATTITUDE! Why not give yourself a new style beginning? Make your style simple, easy, and effortless with these resolutions based on what you've just learned about in this style book.

1. Say yes to a dress.

Step up your style with a dress. They are the easiest way to put an outfit together—just put it on and you're ready to go!

2. Accept that perfection doesn't exist.

There isn't a woman in the world who believes she has the perfect body. Luckily we have clothes! Choose clothes with great fit and you'll forget about your imperfections.

3. Dump the deadbeats.

You wear only 20% of the clothing you own. The other 80% is taking up valuable real estate in your closet. Edit your closet and keep only what you love to wear.

4. Embrace color.

Any wardrobe can be revived with a little bit of color. Not sure what colors look right on you? Remember that one color exists in many different shades. Hold a color up to your face in order to judge which shade is right for you.

5. Give a shout out to shoes.

The easiest way to change the look of an outfit is to simply change your shoes. Shoes are a great way to express the personality of your style.

6. Be willing to try ANYTHING on.

Remember that clothes are meant to be fun so why not have an open mind and try anything on. If you don't like something, just take it off.

7. Shop smart.

When in doubt about what to buy calculate its cost per wear. Divide the cost of the item by the number of times it can potentially be worn to find out whether or not it will be a good investment for you.

8. Dress the body you have right NOW.

Does your style reflect who you are today—body, mind, and lifestyle? Your style tells the world who you are so be sure you know what your clothes are saying.

9. **Think about proportion.**

Dress your body in the most flattering way by paying attention to your body proportion. Aim to balance the proportion of your top and bottom half. For example, if you have broad shoulders choose an a-line skirt to balance out your bottom half.

10. **Try something new.**

Style like life constantly evolves. Keep your style fun and fresh by trying something new. It can be as easy as trying a red shoe, a patterned top, or a bold necklace.

Make sure your closet has these style essentials!

Jackets

€   Denim Jacket

€   Leather Jacket

€   Trench Coat

€   Casual Cotton Twill Jacket/Neutral Color.

Color: _____

€   _____

€   _____

Jeans

€   Dark Denim Jean hemmed for heels

€   Dark/Medium Wash jean hemmed for flats

€   White Jean

€   _____

€   _____

Trousers

€   3 pairs of neutral year round weight trousers

Color 1:_____

Color 2:_____

Color 3:_____

Tops

€   Printed Blouse

€   3 Solid Blouses, Rich colors/varying necklines

Color/Neckline:_____

Color/Neckline:_____

Color/Neckline:_____

€   White Top

€   Fitted white tee (for layering)

€   Fitted black tee (for layering)

€   Fitted grey tee (for layering)

Dresses

€   Black Dress

€   Solid Colored Dress

Color:_____

€   Printed Dress

Print Colors:_____

Skirts

€   Casual Skirt (Denim, Cotton, Etc.)

Color:_____

€   Classic Skirt (solid colored A-line or Pencil)

Color:_____

Shoes

€   Ballet Flat

€   Knee High boots in black / brown

€   Black Heels

€   Brown Heels

€ Sandal

€ Nude shoe (heel, wedge, flat, or sandal)

€ Fun Shoe (Pop of color, embellishment, print)

Purses

€ Black Bag

€ Brown Bag

€ Fun color or printed bag

€ Clutch

Down Undies

€ Convertible Nude Bra

€ Camisoles or Bandeaux for modesty layering

€ Seamless panties in Nude

€ Shaping undergarments

Accessories

€ Stud Earrings

€ Large bold earrings

€ Long necklace

€ Short necklace (great if long & short can be layered together)

€ Bold chunky necklace in pseudo-neutral color

€ Watch (not sporty)

€ Scarf in fun print and color

€ 3 belts (neutral belt to wear with trousers, neutral belt to wear at your waist, Waist belt with pop of color)

My Own Style Notes: